PANDEMIC INFLUENZA
1700–1900

PANDEMIC INFLUENZA
1700–1900

A Study in Historical Epidemiology

K. DAVID PATTERSON

ROWMAN & LITTLEFIELD
Publishers

ROWMAN & LITTLEFIELD

Published in the United States of America in 1986
by Rowman & Littlefield, Publishers
(a division of Littlefield, Adams & Company)
81 Adams Drive, Totowa, New Jersey 07512

Library of Congress Cataloging-in-Publication Data

Patterson, K. David (Karl David), 1941–
  Pandemic influenza, 1700–1900.

  Includes index.
  1. Influenza—Epidemiology—History. 2. Epidemics
—History. I. Title. [DNLM: 1. Disease Outbreaks—
history. 2. Disease Outbreaks—occurrence.
3. Influenza—history. 4. Influenza—occurrence.
WC 515 P317p]
RC150.4.P38 1986   614.5′18′09   86-21903
ISBN 0-8476-7512-2

89 88 87 86
6 5 4 3 2 1

Printed in the United States of America

FOR JEN, DOUG, DANNY, AND KOLA

Contents

Tables

Figures

Maps

Introduction

Influenza is a major cause of sickness and death around the world and is one of the most important infectious diseases confronting the United States and other developed countries. Combined with pneumonia, influenza is one of the ten leading causes of death in the United States. Even though most of its victims are elderly, pneumonia-influenza is the only infectious condition listed in the top ten causes of years of potential life lost by the Centers for Disease Control. These facts, plus the memory of the great pandemic of 1918–1919, which killed about 550,000 people in the United States and claimed over 20 million lives around the world, have encouraged a great deal of research on the flu. The origins of virulent strains and the behavior of epidemics are still not well understood, however, and the unpredictability of influenza presents serious problems for public health planners.

Research on past epidemics has both historical and epidemiological significance. The 1918–1919 pandemic, the most devastating outbreak of infectious disease since the plague swept Asia and Europe in the fourteenth century, has attracted the attention of many historians, but very few have looked at earlier epidemics. Biomedical writers have sometimes used historical data to study the etiology and epidemiology of diseases, and in this tradition prominent students of influenza, such as Vaughan, Kilbourne, and Beveridge, have looked to the past for clues to the behavior of influenza. None of the pre-1918 epidemics has been adequately described, however. The few old compilations available, such as those by Creighton, Finkler, Ripperger, Symes-Thompson, Thompson, and especially Hirsch, have lasting value but are far from infallible, do not invariably consider all relevant data, and are the product of a very different intellectual environment. Modern accounts based on these same authorities represent, from an historian's viewpoint, a rather amateurish and uncritical use of secondary sources. Much of what we think we know may turn out to be erroneous but oft-repeated nineteenth-century opinions.

My objective in this work is to examine eighteenth and nineteenth-century influenza outbreaks in detail, using primary sources whenever possible and asking questions based on modern knowledge. Places of origin of epidemics and the geography of their spread will be described and mapped. Since true pandemics are marked by major antigenic shifts, distinguishing between epidemics and pandemics of the past gives a measure of how often a novel and potentially serious viral strain is likely to emerge. Morbidity and mortality patterns will be discussed and, when possible, quantified. Early observations on seasonality, climatic associations, possible herald waves, and links with flulike illnesses among animals are relevant to modern epidemiological concerns, as are the influences of changes in socioeconomic conditions. Our understanding of influenza is mostly derived from the post-1918 period; accurate knowledge of the past will provide a fuller understanding of the range of behavior of influenza and allow us to assess the tragedy of 1918 in better perspective. Study of early epidemics will not resolve all current mysteries about influenza or any other disease, but historical epidemiology can make a contribution if and only if it is based on sound scholarship.

It is a pleasure to thank the institutions and individuals who have assisted my research. Financial support from the Southern Regional Education Board, the National Endowment for the Humanities Travel to Collections Program, and the Foundation of the University of North Carolina at Charlotte enabled me to conduct much of the research for the first half of the nineteenth century. A preliminary version of some of the material presented in chapter 3 of this work was previously published as "Pandemic and Epidemic Influenza, 1830–1848," in *Social Science and Medicine* 21, no. 5 (1985): 571–80. A Reassignment of Duties Leave from UNCC for spring semester, 1985, and Grant 1 RO1 LM04225-01 from the National Library of Medicine for the fall semester were essential to the completion of this project.

Much of the research was conducted at the Francis A. Countway Library of Medicine in Boston and the National Library of Medicine in Bethesda, Maryland. Special thanks are due to Mr. Richard J. Wolfe at the Countway and Dr. James Cassedy at the NLM. Dr. Gerald F. Pyle of the Geography Department at the University of North Carolina, Charlotte, first encouraged me to extend my interest in influenza from Africa to the rest of the world; I am grateful to him for continuing intellectual, practical, and moral support. This volume is in many ways complementary to his book *The Diffusion of Influenza: Patterns and Paradigms* (Rowman & Littlefield, 1986). Sources for this study are in several European languages, and I am indebted to several people for essential linguistic assistance. My mother, Mrs.

Elizabeth C. Patterson, translated all of the Swedish. Colleagues at UNCC have also been generous with their help. Dr. Janet Levy translated Danish and gave archaeological advice, Dr. Jane Laurent aided with Italian, and Dr. Martha L. Miller did the same with Spanish. Dr. Robert W. Rieke deserves special credit for helping me wade through a large amount of German. Dr. Ann Jannetta of the University of Pittsburg supplied flu data from Japanese sources she is using in her research on the history of disease in that country, and Dr. Frank Barrett of York University clarified questions on the history of disease mapping. Sarah Park Stuart of the UNCC Cartography Laboratory prepared the maps and figures. Finally, I must thank Mary Bottomly and Connie Higginbotham, secretaries in the Department of History, for their able and gracious labor in preparing the manuscript. Gratitude to others does not, of course, absolve me from full responsibility for any errors or omissions.

K. David Patterson
Charlotte, North Carolina

1
The Virus and the Disease

Influenza, an acute viral disease that has afflicted man for centuries, remains one of the most important infectious diseases in the wealthier countries of the world. Flu is a major cause of sickness and, especially among the elderly, a significant cause of death. In conjunction with pneumonia, influenza is the only infectious disease among the top ten killers in the United States, both in terms of numbers of deaths and years of potential life lost.[1] Extensive vaccination campaigns are conducted annually in many countries among the elderly and other vulnerable segments of the population, partly because of the public health importance of the disease, and partly because of the legacy of 1918.

Memories of the catastrophic pandemic of fall-winter 1918–1919 have conditioned all subsequent research and policy on influenza. Influenza epidemics had raged before, most notably in the great pandemic of 1889–1890, but the second or fall wave that swept the world near the end of World War I was totally unprecedented. An estimated 550,000 people died in the United States,[2] about ten times the number of American battle deaths in the war. The most widely cited estimate of the worldwide total is Jordan's estimate of about 21 million.[3] This figure is almost certainly too low as, for example, deaths in Africa were 150 to 200 percent greater than Jordan thought,[4] and he had no figures at all for China. Indeed, a prominent student of the disease has suggested that influenza was responsible for 50 to 100 million deaths, an estimate that seem high, but is certainly possible.[5] In any case, roughly 200 to 300 percent as many people died because of influenza in six months than perished in military actions in more than four years of what was up to then the most devastating war in human history. In addition to its overall mortality, the 1918 pandemic was unique in causing higher death rates among young adults than among the elderly. A virulent strain of influenza virus, acting in conjunction with severe bacterial pneumonias, caused the most deadly epidemic in modern world history. Only the plague that swept Asia, the Middle East, and Europe in the mid-14th century killed more people.

Two great questions have run through thinking about influenza in the last few decades. The first is, what causes a pandemic? The viral etiology of the disease was established in the early 1930s but, despite considerable progress we still cannot fully explain the origins of pandemics, let alone predict where or when one will start. The second question is whether something like 1918 could happen again. We do not know. Indeed, while the identity of the 1918 strain seems to have been established as a "swine flu" (H1N1), we still have no generally accepted explanation of why it was so deadly.[6]

Influenza is caused by an orthomyxovirus. The type called influenza A causes pandemics and will be the focus of this study; influenza B and C viruses are much less epidemiologically important. The influenza A genome consists of eight separate pieces of single-stranded RNA. These eight segments function as distinct genes, so genetic reassortment occurs readily when a host cell is infected with two strains of virus. Such reassortments are genetically equivalent to recombinations and are, as will be described below, a major source of the virus's remarkable antigenic variation. Two of the viral genes code for surface glycoproteins, hemagglutinin (H) and neuraminidase (N), the crucial antigens against which the host develops immunological defenses in the form of circulating antibodies. Thirteen H and nine N subtypes have been discovered,[7] of which H1, H2, H3, N1, and N2 have been positively linked to epidemics in man. Between major epidemics, mutations produce minor but cumulative evolution of antigenic variants within the major H and N subtypes, which seem to help the virus adapt to host immunological defenses. Major new viral subtypes have appeared in 1918, 1957, and 1968, in each case resulting in a pandemic. The term "pandemic" literally means a worldwide epidemic, but for influenza there is also the assumption that a major subtype involving new H and/or N antigens has appeared.[8] These "shifts" are much more dramatic than the normal slow genetic "drift" of prevailing subtypes and, as there has been no (or at least no recent) opportunity for people to develop immunity, the new virus may spread very rapidly. New, potentially pandemic strains probably arise from recombination with viruses from animal reservoirs. A wide range of virus subtypes has been discovered in wild and domesticated animals, most notably pigs, horses, turkeys, and ducks. Feral and domesticated ducks harbor an enormous array of antigenic types and may play a major role in the ecology of the influenza A virus.[9] In this century there have been four major shifts: 1918 (Hsw1N1 = H1N1), 1957 (H2N2), 1968 (H3N2), and a very puzzling reappearance of a 1950 strain of H1N1, which began to circulate again in 1977.[10] There is some evidence that only a limited number of antigenic types recirculate over time in man. Immunological studies of elderly persons suggest that the 1889 pandemic was probably caused by an H2 virus and that the apparent minor pandemic of around 1900 may have been associated with an H3 virus.[11]

Influenza is transferred from person to person by the respiratory route, so human behavior and mobility are crucial factors in the epidemiology of the disease. The short incubation period (24 to 72 hours) facilitates rapid transmission, especially of antigenically novel strains. In temperate latitudes epidemics usually occur in winter, although summer outbreaks are not unknown. Thus, the Northern and Southern Hemispheres often experience influenza six months apart. The reasons for this seasonality are not clear, but cool, dry air seems to favor the survival of the virus in the environment. Human behavior is also significant. People tend to congregate indoors in cold weather, and a high enough percentage of children attended school by the late nineteenth century to make the academic calendar very relevant to flu transmission. Seasonality is less evident in the tropics, although the spread of influenza in parts of Africa in 1918 may have been faster when it coincided with the dry season.[12]

Influenza epidemics are generally characterized by high morbidity and low case-mortality, with highest death rates among the elderly. Most deaths follow secondary pneumonia and/or chronic health problems. The pattern in 1918, with relatively high case-mortality and a remarkable excess death rate for young adults, seems to have been exceptional.

The definition of a pandemic presents major difficulties in the pre-1889 period. Obviously there can be no direct evidence of a new viral type, so other criteria must be adopted. Prior to 1492, potentially pandemic strains must have been restricted to their hemispheres of origin. Between the start of what Crosby has so aptly dubbed the "Columbian Exchange"[13] and the transportation revolution of the mid-nineteenth century, some potentially pandemic strains probably did not have the opportunity for global circulation. Flu usually would die out for lack of new victims after sweeping crews of sailing ships on long voyages. Even if the virus did manage to spread over the world, the patchy nature of surviving records might not reveal it. Not until the 1889–1890 pandemic, when railroads and steamships were available to transport man and virus, can we document a truly worldwide pandemic. For purposes of this study, an influenza pandemic will be defined as a very widespread outbreak with high morbidity, which spread rapidly in a definite pattern as though from a common origin, and which appeared to contemporary observers to be a new and sudden epidemic. Wide and rapid diffusion with extensive morbidity will serve as a measure of the high infectivity expected with pandemic strains. Since infectivity is not necessarily linked to pathogenicity,[14] high mortality is not a criterion, even though a virulent virus might be more easily propagated.

Influenza has been extensively monitored since 1918, and much has been learned about its epidemiology. Over the last few decades powerful techniques from virology, immunology, and molecular biology have produced important new knowledge. Modern biomedical tools have been available, however, for only a very short portion of man's experience with influenza. Historical study of pre-1918 epidemics can give evidence of the disease's occurrence and impact over a much longer period of time, permitting a fuller appreciation of the range of possible behaviors of epidemics and enabling us to put recent episodes into a broader context. While we obviously cannot fully apply modern scientific techniques to events of past centuries, sound historical study can extend our epidemiological experience. We can, for example, attempt to determine the frequency of pandemics and, hence, the frequency of major viral shifts. The past can yield information on the origins and modes of diffusion of pandemics, as well as data on seasonality, weather, animal associations, herald waves, and human activities that might shed light on current theories. For example, it is possible that knowledge of diffusion and morbidity-mortality patterns will shed some light on the theory of H-N antigen recycling, especially for periods too early for serological investigation. Of course, a successful new virus must appear at a specific place and time, so a pandemic has a specific origin. Today there is considerable speculation and some evidence to suggest southern China as an epicenter for new pandemic strains; indeed, the 1957, 1968, and 1977 pandemics did originate in China.[15] Many earlier writers tended to look to Russia or Central Asia as the birthplace of epidemics.[16] Historical analysis should shed some light on this problem. Finally, information on past morbidity and mortality, while necessarily based on a weak statistical base, will illustrate how significant a public health problem influenza can be and will help put the disaster of 1918 into a wider context.

Epidemiologists, virologists, and other influenza researchers have frequently examined the historical record for clues to the present and future behavior of the disease. Most discussions of influenza epidemiology draw upon the pre-1918 period, at least in passing, for evidence on the origins, periodicity, diffusion, and morbidity-mortality patterns of the disease.[17] Historians, on the other hand, have been mesmerized by the drama of 1918 and have devoted little attention to earlier events.[18] Most of what has been written on influenza in previous centuries has been sketchy and has not been based on primary sources. Instead, accounts have been drawn from a handful of nineteenth-century German and English compilers, notably August Hirsch, Charles Creighton, Theophilus Thompson, and A. Ripperger. These authors in turn have used such early nineteenth-century writers as J.A.F. Ozanam, Heinrich Schweich, and Gottlieb Gluge, as well as contemporary accounts. They have pulled together a great deal of literature and presented it in convenient form. Despite the collective virtues of Hirsch and the others, however, real research must go beyond such secondary sources. Clearly, if historical epidemiology is to provide useful information, it must be based on sound historical methodology. These standard and some lesser-known nineteenth-century authorities are freely used in this study, but I go beyond them in two ways. First, I have consulted as much primary material as possible. I have located many sources not consulted by the nineteenth-century compilers and, in many other cases, have been able to correct erroneous interpretations that have crept into their works. Second, modern knowledge and current problems allow new questions to be framed on the basis of the older material.

The early history of influenza, like that of virtually all diseases, is shrouded in mystery. Since it does not occur among apes,[19] influenza apparently is not part of our primate heritage. Indeed, as an acute infection that does not have a latent phase in people, its survival depends on the existence of large numbers of susceptible victims in frequent contact with each other. Like many infectious diseases, influenza could not have been more than a sporadic infection in man until the development of agriculture and the growth of towns.[20] Yet because of the great antigenic variability of the influenza virus, the disease can maintain itself in much smaller populations than, for example, measles or smallpox. Influenza could therefore be one of the older viral diseases of man. In any case, it is reasonable to assume that the influenza virus evolved in birds and/or mammals and then became established in humans, perhaps after several abortive attempts, and perhaps independently in more than one place, no earlier than several millennia B.C.

Where influenza first became established as a human disease is of course unknown, but it was presumably in one of the four regions of the ancient world that McNeil has postulated as the "civilized disease pools of Eurasia." These relatively densely populated areas —northern China, northern India, the Middle East, and the eastern Mediterranean—were all early centers of agricultural and urban life.[21] It is entirely possible that the advent of human influenza was connected with the domestication of animals. Among the animals implicated today as possible reservoir hosts, pigs were domesticated in both China and the Middle East by circa 5000 B.C. and spread to the other regions quite quickly; horses were widely used by circa 1500–2000 B.C., and ducks were being raised in the Middle East by circa 2500 B.C., and in China by circa 2000 B.C. and perhaps much earlier.[22]

It is just conceivable that, given the wide-ranging travels of some Arctic peoples, influenza accompanied or was carried to the ancestors of modern Indian and/or Eskimo populations across the Bering Strait, but low population densities in northeast Asia make this unlikely. It is also possible that feral ducks or other migratory birds introduced influenza A viruses to Amerindian populations prior to European contact. Population densities in central and southern Mexico and in the Andean highlands were certainly high enough to sustain viral circulation, and the Moscovy duck had been domesticated by the early inhabitants of Peru. There is, however, no evidence that influenza existed in the Americas in the pre-Columbian period, and it was almost certainly introduced by the Spanish and/or other Europeans in the early sixteenth-century.

Epidemics of influenza must have been fairly frequent in ancient and medieval times, but not until 1173 was one described well enough to allow a scholar, Hirsch, to determine that the disease was in fact influenza.[23] Other writers are more cautious; Ripperger, for example, was not confident enough about early accounts to decide on a definite diagnosis of influenza until 1387.[24] These and other writers list several widespread outbreaks in the fifteenth and sixteenth centuries, with especially large epidemics, perhaps pandemics, recorded in 1510, 1557, and 1580. In 1580 influenza swept northward from the Mediterranean to the Baltic in four months in what was probably a true pandemic.[25] There were several regional European outbreaks of influenza in the seventeenth century, but apparently nothing resembling a pandemic.[26]

This study focuses on the 1700–1900 period for very pragmatic reasons. Documentation on pre-eighteenth century epidemics is scanty and, with very few exceptions, difficult to locate in this country. Despite some real problems in quantity and quality of materials, especially in the first half of the 1700s, there is sufficient information for fairly complete descriptions and meaningful analysis of eighteenth-century and nineteenth-century events. The possible pandemic of circa 1900 will be discussed, but no attempt will be made to add to the voluminous but still inadequate literature on 1918.

Although influenza has been given dozens of names over the centuries, nomenclature is not a serious problem for this period. Popular terms have ranged from the fanciful (jolie rant, gallant, sheep's cough) to ascriptions of origin (Russian catarrh, Chinese flu, Scottish rant). The geographical tradition has, of course, continued into this century, with the "Asian" flu of 1957, the "Hong Kong" flu of 1968, and the misleading label of "Spanish" flu for 1918. Current rules require that new strains of viruses include their place of isolation as part of their official names (for example, A/Brazil/11/78). Older terms like "epidemic catarrh" were frequently used up to the mid-nineteenth century. The word "influenza" was introduced into English from Italian in 1743 and has since become the most common medical term in English, German, and most other European languages. The French have used "grippe" since the mid-eighteenth century; Belgian, Spanish, and Portuguese writers have usually followed their example. This terminological dichotomy caused no confusion; "influenza" and "grippe" were used interchangeably by some authors and were universally understood to be synonyms.[27]

The existing sources inevitably shape and limit this or any other historical study. Eighteenth- and nineteenth-century information is geographically uneven, with data most abundant by far for Western Europe, notably Britain, Germany, France, and northern Italy. Scandinavia, Russia, the Iberian Peninsula, and especially the Balkans are more sparsely documented in the contemporary medical literature, but we can usually construct a fairly satisfactory picture of influenza activity in Europe. Reports on Asia, the Middle East, Africa, and South America are sketchy at best and usually supplied by European observers. North American data are better, but often quite disappointing. Given the skewed geographical coverage of the medical literature, much of the evidence presented here of necessity focuses on Europe. It must be stressed that the absence of reports from a particular region during an epidemic does not necessarily mean that influenza did not occur there.

The sources present many other problems. Eighteenth- and nineteenth-century medical writers had their own concerns and were not always aware of or able to provide the kinds of data of interest to twentieth-century readers. For example, much energy was devoted to lengthy and sometimes heated arguments over whether influenza was caused and/or spread by atmospheric poisons or miasmas, meteorological phenomena, telluric factors such as volcanoes or earthquakes, or by person-to-person contagion. Miasmatists were generally less likely to present geographical data than the contagionists. Debates over whether influenza was a discrete disease or just a variant or an early stage or sequel of catarrh, pneumonia, or some other disease take up a substantial portion of many articles. For example, the great cholera epidemic that swept Europe and North America in 1831–1832 stimulated extensive speculation that the 1831 influenza was somehow a precursor of cholera, or that cholera prepared the way for the influenza epidemic of 1833. Many less theoretical articles, whose titles looked promising when first encountered, turned out to be repetitious compilations of case histories. In order to understand the literature fully, some attention will have to be devoted to the evolution of medical views and practices concerning influenza.

Geographical reconstruction of the spread of epidemics is often hampered because contemporary observers often reported the dates when the disease appeared in a given place in a very vague manner. Most frequently they mentioned a month, not a particular day or week. More specific times are sometimes reported ("toward the end of October"), but even then accounts of when an epidemic began or prevailed can be misleading. Authors may cite the first scattered and perhaps unrelated cases, the first cases that were clearly part of the epidemic wave, or impressions of the morbidity or mortality peaks. Another difficulty is that since many eighteenth- and nineteenth-century writers did not view influenza as an entity capable of moving over space, they did not attempt to describe paths of spread. Maps had been used in studies of yellow fever in the 1790s and of cholera in the mid-nineteenth century, but I have found no attempts to map influenza prior to 1889.[28] Consequently, diffusion patterns usually must be inferred from static accounts of places and dates.

For most of the period under consideration, information on morbidity and mortality was mostly impressionistic and at best fragmentary, given the primitive state of both diagnosis and vital statistics. Vital statistics were systematically reported in most of Europe by the late nineteenth century, but most states in the United States and most of the rest of the world did not collect or publish such data. Even when mortality figures were based on numbers of burials or on official returns, as in Britain from the 1840s and even earlier in some localities, there are severe methodological problems. Even now it is difficult to measure the effect of influenza on mortality. Influenza was, and still is, sometimes given as the cause of death, but in most cases the disease is fatal only when complicated with secondary bacterial pneumonias and/or when it attacks persons with severe chronic diseases. Criteria for assigning causes of death vary now and have varied widely in the past with changes in medical knowledge and with local customs and laws. The Centers for Disease Control publish a combined pneumonia-influenza death tally as an index of influenza activity, but this index, also employed in the nineteenth century, may understate the total impact of the disease.[29] Another useful index of influenza activity, used by the pioneering English health statistician William Farr in the 1840s and widely employed since then, is total "excess" mortality. That is, in the absence of other known factors, deaths above the average during a period of influenza activity are assumed to be related to the epidemic.[30] Figures for total deaths are often available when cause-specific data cannot be found, and this measure will be used often in this study, especially in the discussion of the 1889–1890 pandemic. Fortunately, mortality returns, whether total or cause-specific, were often published by sex and age.

Morbidity is even harder to measure, since so many cases are mild or never come to the attention of a doctor. Even today, with sample interview surveys, returns from clinics and institutional populations, reports from sentinel physicians, virological and immunological surveys, and compilation of data on absenteeism from schools and workplaces, morbidity rates are far from precise. For earlier centuries, the only measures are the guesses of informed observers as to what fraction of a locality's population got sick.

Two other problems with the older sources deserve mention. Accurate diagnosis is a general problem for historians of disease, and is a real issue for sporadic cases and the early phases of influenza epidemics. There is no difficulty in recognizing major epidemics, however, at least by the eighteenth century. Observers knew what they were dealing with and frequently made comparisons with earlier epidemics. The pervasive xenogenic assumption that epidemics always came from somewhere else, usually eastward, may bias some accounts; a few authors, such as the otherwise very useful Gluge,[31] may have tried too hard to fit data into a preconceived framework of east-to-west diffusion. Our knowledge of past epidemics will always be incomplete, with major issues often unresolved and many conclusions tentative. Sero-archeology can shed some light on the late nineteenth century but, unless old serum specimens have somehow survived and can be analyzed, it will be impossible to connect, distinguish between, or virologically characterize earlier pandemics with any degree of certainty. We can, however, learn a lot that goes beyond our present hazy knowledge of this intrinsically historical disease.

In sum, the goals of this study are to make critical use of the best historical sources for the eighteenth and nineteenth centuries in the light of modern knowledge in order to extend our epidemiological understanding of pandemic influenza. Several questions will be asked. How often did pandemics occur? Where did they originate, and how did they spread? What impact has influenza had on public health, as measured by both morbidity and mortality? How have medical views and tactics been influenced by epidemiological experience, and how have physicians' beliefs influenced their opinions? Finally, can analysis of morbidity, mortality, and geographical diffusion patterns, in conjunction with serological studies, allow us to make comparisons between twentieth-century and earlier pandemics and shed light on the antigen recycling theory?

2
Influenza in the Eighteenth Century

The world of the eighteenth century was obviously very different from our own in many epidemiologically significant ways. As most of the data on influenza in that century comes from Western Europe, some general statements on conditions there are in order. Europe's population, something in the order of 120 to 180 million, was much less dense than today. Although cities were growing rapidly, most Europeans still lived in farming villages or in small towns. People did not move around very much. When they did travel, they usually did not go very far, moving only as fast as they or a horse could walk or a boat could sail. Highways and canals improved over the century, especially in Britain and France, but travel remained slow and arduous. Influenza could travel only where and as fast as people could. Cities were then, as now, foci of disease dissemination into the hinterlands, and we may assume that influenza reached urban areas along the trade routes.

The eighteenth-century medical profession was in many ways ill-equipped to deal with influenza.[1] Most doctors recognized the disease as a distinct entity during epidemics, but sporadic cases and those occurring early or late in an epidemic tended to merge into an ill-defined category of colds, catarrhs, and other respiratory complaints and "fevers." Many thought that atmospheric changes, either meteorological or more subtle "atmospheric constitutions," could change simple catarrhs or other fevers into epidemic influenza or vice versa. There was, of course, no concept of viruses and, although "germ" theories had ebbed and flowed in popularity since the mid-1500s, few eighteenth-century observers thought that any type of living agent was responsible for influenza. Instead, some sort of poisonous substance or particle seemed to fit the facts better.[2]

For most doctors, especially in the first six or seven decades of the century, influenza seemed to be spread by, or created by, atmospheric factors. Such theories were complex and quite intellectually respectable, given the state of knowledge of the day. They usually invoked an unknown poison or miasma carried in the air and/or specific winds, temperature changes, barometric pressures, or other meterological factors to explain the appearance and spread of epidemic diseases like influenza. This is why eighteenth- and early nineteenth-century articles on influenza are much more likely to contain elaborate meteorological tables than geographical reconstructions or statistics on morbidity or mortality. On the other hand, diseases like smallpox and syphilis seemed to be spread by close contact, and some physicians—the "contagionists"—took the view that many or most other diseases were spread by transmission of some poison or other agent directly from person to person. Compromise positions between "miasmatists" and "contagionists" were common; "contingent contagionists" could and did argue over how specific diseases were spread, atmospheric influences on contagions, what exactly was meant by person-to-person contact, whether modes of transmission could change during an epidemic, or if and under what conditions some diseases might spread by more than one mechanism. Again, it must be stressed that the evidence was inadequate and ambiguous at best, and it is misleading to label contagionists, who temporarily became more numerous in the 1780s, as necessarily more progressive or better scientists than those who disagreed with them.

Therapy in the eighteenth and early nineteenth centuries was still largely based on humoral ideas derived from classical times,[3] although major new, competing theories of disease etiology and pathology were being advanced in Edinburgh and other medical centers. Treatment was generally based on the idea that in illness the whole body became somehow unbalanced, and many remedies were designed to get rid of noxious substances and directly or indirectly to restore a healthy balance of fluids. Hence the popularity of treatments for a wide range of conditions based on some combination of purges, bleeding, sweating, inducing vomiting or urination, or the production of local blisters as "counterirritants." Most doctors recognized that influenza was usually a self-limiting disease and, if they prescribed anything at all beyond bed rest, fluids, "cordial" spirits, or quinine (as a "tonic" and/or febrifuge), they generally employed only mild purges, emetics, or less commonly, bleeding. Many warned against vigorous measures, which would only further debilitate the patient. Much more extensive and harmful measures, particularly bleeding, were sometimes used when pneumonia developed, but even in acute cases there was much controversy over what to do and how far to go. In general, despite stereotypes of excessive bleeding and purging, most doctors employed quite sensible therapeutic regimes for influenza.

Influenza pandemics occurred at least three times in the eighteenth century: 1729–1730, 1732–1733, and 1781–1782. In addition, there were two major epidemics that could possibly be considered pandemics, in 1761–1762 and 1788–1789, and at least eight other notable epidemics during the century.[4] The number and quality of the sources for these outbreaks is very uneven. There is much more information for 1781–1782 than for any other period, but even for that major pandemic, quantitative data are very sparse. Morbidity estimates are guesses, and mortality is known only from scattered church burial lists or, in a few places, totals compiled with varying degrees of care by municipal governments. There is a strong geographical bias in the literature toward western Europe and especially Britain, for which data are much more abundant than, for example, the Balkans or North America. The sources are good enough to create a general picture of the epidemiology of influenza in the eighteenth century, but many major questions cannot be answered unless new records are discovered.

The first influenza epidemic of the eighteenth century took place in 1708–1709. According to contemporary accounts, which are sparse, the disease was apparently restricted to western Europe.[5] The first outbreak was in Rome around Christmas of 1708. The disease spread to northern Italy in January and February 1709, to France and Belgium in March, Berlin in April, and Denmark sometime in the summer. Much of Germany was attacked, as was Laibach (Ljubljana) in what is now northern Yugoslavia, but the Iberian Peninsula was apparently spared, and it is not clear whether influenza reached Norway and Sweden. Ireland was affected, but England probably was not. This epidemic, while locally severe, was not a true pandemic. The apparent north to south spread, reminiscent of the 1580 pandemic, is quite unusual.

Another extensive but nonpandemic episode took place in 1712.[6] The epidemic began in central Germany, with first reports from Jena in April. Copenhagen and the German regions of Thuringia and Saxony were involved by late May or early June, Holstein in July, Bavaria and Holland in August, Württemberg in southwest Germany in September, and northern Italy in December. There is no record of influenza in France, England, Spain, or eastern Europe at this time. Although morbidity was very high and observers considered the epidemic more severe than the 1709 episode, the limited geographical extent of the epidemic strongly indicates that there was no new pandemic strain. The summertime spread is notable.

A major pandemic occurred in 1729–1730 (see Map 2.1).[7] Initial reports were of substantial outbreaks in two widely separated Russian cities, Moscow and Astrakhan, on the Caspian Sea in April 1729. There were no further reports during the summer, but influ-

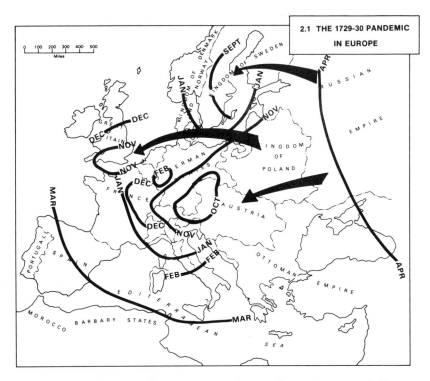

2.1 THE 1729-30 PANDEMIC IN EUROPE

enza prevailed in Sweden in September and in Vienna and Upper
Silesia in October. During November flu was prevalent in Hungary
and Poland,[8] swept deep into Germany and appeared in London,
Plymouth, York, and Durham[9] in England, as well as in Dublin.[10] In
December flu attacked Scotland, several Swiss cities and, at the end
of the month, Paris.[11] So many monks fell ill in the French capital
that the monasteries had to cancel religious services. Northern Italy,
including Padua and Bologna, was attacked in January 1730, Rome
and the Papal States in February,[12] and Naples, Sicily, and Spain in
March. Also in March, Iceland began to experience its first fully
documented influenza epidemic. The disease was introduced into
the south, probably at Reykjavik, and spread northward over the
island.[13]

   The 1729–1730 pandemic may have become truly worldwide. Flu
apparently did not break out in North America until October 1732,[14]
when the disease was widespread along the New England coast from
Boston to southern Maine. By November it was active in New York,
Philadelphia, and New Jersey. It seems not to have spread as far
south as South Carolina,[15] but in October it was said to be prevalent
in such widely separated places as Newfoundland, Jamaica, Mexico,

Barbados, and Peru.[16] Influenza with high morbidity was reported on the remote French island of Bourbon (Réunion) in the Indian Ocean at the end of 1732.[17]

Although the origins and termination of the 1729–1730 episode are unclear, it obviously was a pandemic, the first of a series that western European observers saw as coming from Russia.[18] An origin in Russia seems very plausible, but there is no documentation of this, and the long silence between April in Moscow and September in Sweden is suspicious. Indeed, it is possible that the Russian strain was distinct from the virus that surfaced in the fall and that, as some authors have suggested, the pandemic really originated in Sweden,[19] diffusing southward into Poland and Germany and, via sea trade, to England. A report of a quite late (November) involvement of Riga,[20] Russia's newly acquired Baltic port, tends to support this hypothesis; but the early reports from Vienna and Silesia make overland transmission westward from Russia seem more likely. While certainty is impossible, especially given the scarcity of data from eastern Europe, the most economical hypothesis is that the epidemic did develop in, or at least spread in European Russia in the early months of 1729. Scattered cases caused early dissemination or "pre-seeding" of the virus among the population of Sweden, and probably in the Ukraine and Poland as well, during the summer. The epidemic broke out in the fall, when conditions were favorable for rapid propagation of the virus, with subsequent diffusion west and south. England's early involvement almost certainly resulted from the Baltic trade.

The epidemic in isolated Réunion probably was a late manifestation of this pandemic, but Western Hemisphere events are much more difficult to interpret. Contemporary accounts are few and laconic, but the sudden October 1732 outbursts from Peru to Newfoundland certainly suggest pre-seeding. On the other hand, if this were true, the extensive trans-Atlantic commerce would have been expected to result in an epidemic in the fall of 1731, rather than a year later. As will be discussed below, most observers have linked this New World influenza to the 1732–1733 pandemic in Europe. It is, of course, entirely possible that events in the Americas were independent of either Old World pandemic.

Quantitive evidence is lacking, but the 1729–1730 pandemic seems to have caused much sickness but relatively few deaths. Morbidity was generally reported to be very extensive,[21] even if a statement that only five out of every thousand residents of Lucerne, Switzerland, escaped infection is surely exaggerated.[22] Mortality was generally low, although case-fatality was considered serious in

Ravenna and Ferrara in northern Italy.[23] In England, parish burial returns show a substantial jump in December 1729, probably due to influenza.[24] Persons of all ages were stricken, but deaths were most numerous among the elderly[25] and, according to one writer, among pregnant women.[26] In terms of morbidity and mortality, as well as in rapid, extensive geographical spread, the influenza outbreak of 1729–1730 was a true pandemic.

Another great pandemic swept Europe from east to west in 1732–1733 (Map 2.2). Thus, as would happen a century later in 1830–1831 and 1833, there were independent pandemics within three years of each other.[27] This pandemic developed, or at least first came to written notice, in Russia, where it was already widespread by November 1732.[28] It spread over Poland to the central German regions of Saxony and Thuringia by the end of the month,[29] and by the end of December influenza had swept across the German lands to Alsace.[30] In December, it also reached Basel, Switzerland, and on the 17th broke out in Edinburgh, Scotland.[31] During January 1733, London, Newcastle, Dublin, Paris, Flanders, and the northern Italian cities of Milan, Verona, and Vicenza were attacked. Leghorn (Livorno) in central Italy and southwestern England, including

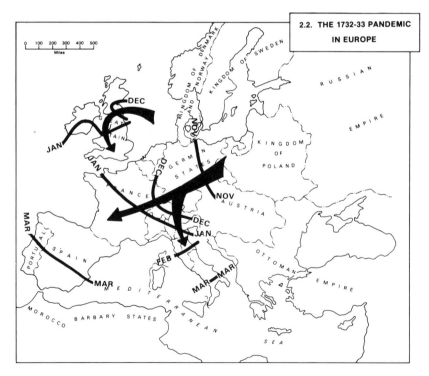

2.2. THE 1732-33 PANDEMIC IN EUROPE

Cornwall, Devonshire, and the port of Plymouth,[32] escaped until February. Madrid and southern Italy (Naples) were attacked in March[33] and the island of Majorca in April.

The east-west course of this pandemic seems clear, even if information on Russia is sparse. Early involvement of Scotland, as in 1729–1730, may well be due to the Baltic trade. London and Paris were both hit in mid-January; London from the north and Paris from the east, with diffusion into the Low Countries probably from both directions.

As discussed earlier, there was extensive influenza activity in North and South America in October and November 1732, at the same time as the disease was moving through Russia and Poland into Germany. The early American compiler Webster wrote that the "universal influenza of 1733 began in America in the autumn of 1732. It appeared in Europe in December."[34] This hypothesis of an American origin is cautiously supported by Fuster,[35] but denied by Gluge[36] and Ripperger.[37] It is certainly possible that the American colonies of Britain exported flu to Europe: sailing time from New England to the mother country was only four to six weeks. December is too early a date for England, and the late involvement of southern England, including Plymouth, a main port for the American trade, argues against this, as does, though less convincingly, the fact that Madrid was spared for so long. While viruses from the New World no doubt eventually did reach Europe, they could not have been there in time to cause the pandemic. Certainly a theory of New World origins could not explain events in eastern and central Europe. The influenza of late 1732 in the Americas probably represents a late flare-up of the 1729–1730 pandemic or, just possibly, an independent epidemic. Influenza was epidemic in Japan in 1733; what relations, if any, existed between this outbreak and the pandemics is unclear.[38]

Information on morbidity and mortality is sketchy for this largely pre-statistical era. Morbidity in 1732–1733 seems to have been high everywhere without regard to age, sex, or economic status,[39] and there is no hint in the literature that exposure to the 1729–1730 virus conveyed any residual immunity. Mortality rates remained low, except among infants, the aged, and consumptives and other chronically ill persons.[40] Few died in Palma, Majorca, a fact attributed to the beneficial action of sea air in diluting the miasma thought to cause the disease. Influenza was more lethal on the mainland in Catalonia.[41] More deaths were recorded in London than during the previous epidemic.[42] Burials in Edinburgh's Greyfriars Churchyard in January 1733, at the height of influenza mortality, were said to be twice as numerous as in the usual January. Apparently, most of the city's dead were buried in that cemetery.[43] The actual returns, shown in Figure 2.1, show a sharp peak in January for adults and, perhaps surprisingly, for children. This unique record gives no ages other than the vague category "children," but it does suggest that while case-mortality rates were probably low in 1732–1733, the overall toll in deaths was not negligible.

There was a minor epidemic in 1737–1738, which involved England, Barbados, and the North American colonies in November and December, and France in January.[44] This episode attracted little contemporary attention and seems of slight importance, although possible transatlantic transmission is of some interest.

The next epidemic of any significance took place in 1742–1743. In January and February there was activity in Germany (Coburg, Koblenz, and Dresden), which may or may not have been related to an October outbreak in Switzerland and northern Italy (Brescia). Influenza spread slowly southward in Italy for the rest of 1742, reaching Milan in November, Rome in January 1743, and Naples and Sicily in February. Meanwhile, it arrived in Paris in February 1743, spread north to Belgium and the Netherlands in March, and reached Plymouth and London in April.[45] This epidemic caused much sickness, but spread very slowly and was restricted to portions of western Europe. It clearly was not a pandemic.

Fig. 2.1 Burials at Greyfriar's, Edinburgh, June 1732–May 1733

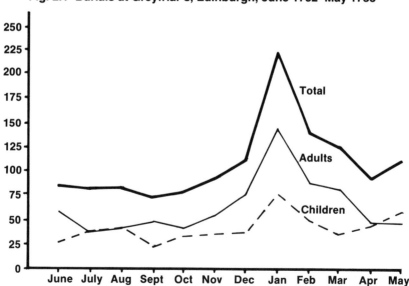

Another apparent minor epidemic with possible origins in North America took place in 1757–1758.[46] Flu was widespread in Britain's mainland colonies and in Barbados in September 1757. The French channel port of Bologne was infected in December, but other French cities like Paris and Lille were not attacked until the following May. Influenza was also active in Scotland and northern England in September and October 1758. Given the scattering of reports, this "epidemic" may well have been just a series of unrelated local outbreaks.

The epidemic of 1761–1762 (Map 2.3) was much more widespread and has sometimes been considered a true pandemic.[47] It occurred toward the end of the Seven Years' War and military movements may have facilitated diffusion of the disease. There are vague reports of flu in North America in early 1761, with Philadelphia involved in the winter, Boston in April, and Barbados in May. These events are probably not related to the European epidemic, which was first reported in Breslau, Silesia (modern Wroclaw) in February 1762. Vienna, Hungary, and Denmark were attacked in March, and by the end of April influenza had covered most of Germany and had reached England, Scotland, and northern Italy.

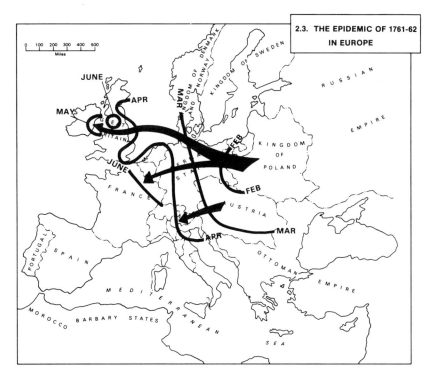

2.3. THE EPIDEMIC OF 1761-62 IN EUROPE

Ireland experienced flu in May, as did rural Cumberland, England. The disease reached Lille and Strasbourg in June and moved south, lingering in parts of France until September. Paris, however, may not have been attacked at all.[48] Morbidity was high in some localities, with an estimate of 90 percent in Vienna,[49] but this epidemic was not seen as particularly severe by contemporary observers. Breslau did experience a sharp rise in mortality during the epidemic.[50] Two geographical factors are worth noting. Although the spread of influenza down the urban hierarchy—that is, from large towns to smaller ones and ultimately to rural villages—must always have been common, this is the first epidemic for which this form of diffusion is explicitly described.[51] Second, although there is no mention of Russia at this time, there is a clear pattern of fairly rapid east-west spread. On the other hand, the epidemic did not attract much comtemporary writing and it seems not to have reached southern Italy or the Iberian or Scandinavian peninsulas. Whether this epidemic was a true pandemic characterized by a major viral shift is unclear; it probably was not, but the case must remain open.

Influenza was epidemic on two other occasions before the great pandemic of the early 1780s. In April 1767 New England and central Germany experienced influenza; London was attacked in June, Lille in July, and Paris in August. Provincial France and Italy were affected during the autumn, and flu reached Madrid and Cayenne, French Guiana, in December.[52] In 1775, influenza was active in Germany and Austria between March and June, appeared in Naples in September, and was widespread in Italy, France, and England from October 1775 through January 1776.[53] Neither of these epidemics seems to have been especially severe, and there were no clear patterns of spread.

Influenza was widely diffused in France[54] and Italy during the first three months of 1780, with an isolated report from Rio de Janeiro, Brazil. In September 1780 flu was noted on the south coast of China (Canton) and in Bengal and on the Coromandel Coast of eastern India.[55] European Russia suffered from influenza during the winter of 1780–1781, as did the United States in the spring of 1781.[56] These events were a prelude to the great pandemic of 1781–1782, but there probably are no direct connections.

The pandemic of 1781–1782 ranks with those of 1889–1890 and 1918–1919 as among the most widespread and dramatic outbreaks of disease in history. It made tens of millions of people sick, spread as rapidly as existing transportation systems permitted and, not surprisingly, attracted a great deal of medical writing. Like its two predecessors a half-century earlier, this pandemic swept Europe from east to west. The earliest reports were from Russia, but for the first time there were suspicions of Asian origins, and there also was contemporary speculation about the role of North America.

Two groups of London physicians formed committees to investigate the epidemic. The committee organized by the Royal College of Physicians learned of an influenza outbreak at Negapatam (Nagappattinam) on the southeastern coast of India in November 1781.[57] The afflicted area was only about a hundred miles south of the Coromandel Coast region, where flu had been active in September 1780. Edward Gray, writing a report of the Society for Promoting Medical Knowledge, learned of influenza in the "East Indies" (presumably modern Indonesia and/or Malaysia) in October and November.[58] The first European reports were from Russia, where influenza was active in Moscow and in Kazan to the east during December 1781.[59] (Map 2.4). British investigators learned that the epidemic had been traced beyond the Urals to Tobolski (Tobolsk), "to which place it was supposed to have been brought from China."[60] St. Petersburg was attacked in January 1782. The disease advanced along both shores of the Baltic in February, moving through southern Finland and to Reval (Tallinn), Riga, and Tilsit and thence into East Prussia

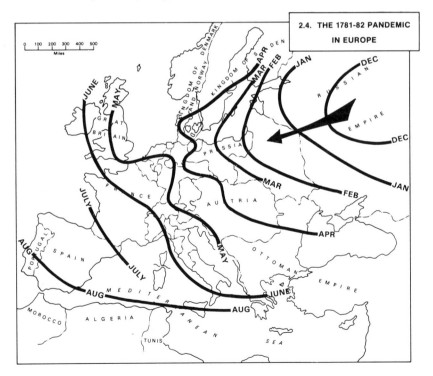

2.4. THE 1781-82 PANDEMIC IN EUROPE

(Braunberg, modern Braunievo, in Poland). During March influenza progressed along the Baltic coast of Germany as far as Pomerania. Influenza exploded across northern Germany in April and reached Hungary (Miskolcz), Denmark (Copenhagen), and Sweden (Stockholm) during the same month. Western Germany, Austria, and Bohemia (Prague) were attacked in May.

London and much of southern England were attacked during the last half of the month, as perhaps was Edinburgh,[61] and at the end of May influenza reached the northern port of Newcastle-upon-Tyne. Several writers, including Hirsch, Ripperger, Finkler, and Pyle and Patterson,[62] relying on the Royal College of Physicians study,[63] have stated that influenza reached Newcastle, its earliest British beachhead, in late April. Yet a detailed report by a local physician, John Clark, shows that Newcastle and its port, Shields, were not infected until late May, probably by sick sailors on ships arriving from London.[64] Clark's date is supported by a doctor writing from nearby Northumberland,[65] so the committee's widely cited version is probably based on a clerical error. London was almost certainly the intitial focus for the British Isles. In any case, influenza spread rapidly over most of England and Scotland during June and crossed the Irish Sea to Dublin by the middle of the month.[66] Diffusion from cities to small towns and rural areas was clearly described for Chester and Durham.[67]

Most of France, the Low Countries, and southwestern Germany were invaded in June. Northern Italy and southern France suffered during July, and the epidemic enveloped southern Italy, Spain, and Portugal during August and September.

European observers carefully noted the spread of disease and were convinced that influenza had come to them from Russia. Popular names like "la Russe,"[68] "catarro russo,"[69] and "russischer Katarrh"[70] clearly expressed this view. The east-west sweep of the pandemic was obvious to all, but several writers thought that its origins lay beyond Russia. As noted above, reports reaching London suggested that the disease reached Russia from China, via western Siberia.[71] A later account notes that Russians had referred to the 1781–1782 influenza by a term equivalent to Chinese catarrh.[72]

Nineteenth-century writers, including Schweich,[73] Haeser,[74] and Martiny,[75] located the origins of the pandemic, respectively, in India, China, or the East Indies, from whence it supposedly spread across "Tartary" and Siberia to European Russia. Japan experienced an epidemic in 1781,[76] which could bolster a theory of Asian origins. The American epidemiologist, lexicographer, and patriot Noah Webster took the whole problem back to the United States. He hypothesized that the epidemic might have started in the spring of 1781 along the Atlantic Coast, from where it spread westward to and over the Pacific to China and "Russian Kamchatka" and thence across Asia to Europe. He admitted that he lacked data to show this,[77] and, although the prominent nineteenth-century French epidemiologist Fuster considered this plausible,[78] it does not seem possible. Webster, a convinced anti-contagionist who believed that atmospheric changes spread epidemics, did not concern himself with transportation systems or population densities. An epidemic spreading from America would certainly have reached western Europe by sea long before it could have reached Asia, let alone Russia. Given the realities of difficult travel conditions over immense distances in sparsely populated territory in North America and Siberia/Central Asia, it seems much more reasonable to suggest that the pandemic strain emerged somewhere in the eastern domains of the Russian Empire, perhaps in western Siberia or the southern Urals. If so, the Asian epidemic(s), vaguely known to us from a few phrases in two British reports, was or were independent events. If the pandemic did in fact originate in Asia, a route from India to Russia via Iran and the Volga seems the most likely, but there is no evidence whatsoever to support such a theory.

The pandemic caused enormous morbidity throughout Europe. Physicians guessed that two-thirds of the population of Rome and three-quarters of the people of Munich fell sick.[79] The overall morbidity in Britain was estimated at 75 to 80 percent.[80] In Exeter, "almost every inhabitant felt its influence,"[81] only one in four remained healthy in Edinburgh,[82] and in Bristol "it was rare for any person to have escaped it."[83] Men and women, rich and poor, the old, middle-aged, and young, all seem equally likely to contract the disease.

Mortality, however, was by all accounts low and generally restricted to the elderly or those with chronic respiratory diseases.[84] Elevated death tolls were reported for both London and Copenhagen,[85] but numerical data are extremely rare. Bills of Mortality for the city of London, presented in Table 2.1, show peaks in total burials and in deaths from "fever" about four weeks after the epidemic began, suggesting that influenza did cause measurable excess mortality. Indeed, although most doctors saw few deaths among their patients, one eminent physician noted that "the bills of mortality . . . seem to speak a different language; and the increase of funerals both in town and country . . . evidently proves that the influenza, or its consequences, occasioned greater fatality than practitioners were aware of."[86]

Table 2.1   London Mortality, 1782

Week	Total burials	Deaths from "fever"
7 May	299	28
14 May	307	34
21 May	336	45
28 May	390	49
4 June	385	57
11 June	560	121
18 June	473	110
25 June	434	89
2 July	296	49

Source: An Account of the Epidemic Disease Called the Influenza of the Year 1782, Collected from the Observations of Several Physicians in London and in the Country, by a Committee of the Fellows of the Royal College of Physicians in London, *"Medical Transactions,"* vol. 3 (London, 1785), 61. These data are also presented as a graph in Richard Sisley, *Epidemic Influenza: Notes on Its Origin and Method of Spread* (London, 1891), 45.

Case-mortality rates were low, but so many people contracted influenza that the total number of deaths in Europe must have been in the hundreds of thousands. There has been a recent assertion that the age distribution of mortality in 1781–1782 resembled that of 1918,[87] when age-specific death rates were remarkably high among young adults. Nevertheless, there is no evidence of any significant deviation from the usual pattern. In 1781–1782 most influenza-related deaths were among the elderly.

The only other significant eighteenth-century outbreak took place in 1788–1789 (Map 2.5). Information is much more sparse than for 1781–1782, and morbidity and mortality seem to have been lower, but some writers have described this epidemic as a possible[88] or actual[89] pandemic. It does present some interesting geographical patterns. The earliest reports were from two Russian cities, St. Petersburg on the Baltic and Kherson, on the Ukrainian coast of the Black Sea, in March 1788.[90] Vienna, Warsaw,[91] and Hungary (Miskolcz) were attacked in April, and there was an isolated account of an outbreak in Eskilstuna, Sweden, beginning in the same month.[92] By the end of May, influenza had reached Copenhagen, and Munich was attacked in June.

Influenza crossed the English Channel in June, striking London late in the month[93] and Plymouth in early July.[94] The epidemic seems to have spread north and west from London, reaching Bath in July and Manchester at the end of the month, where its appearance was blamed on the arrival of sick travelers from London.[95] Scotland (including Aberdeen)[96] and Cornwall were affected in August, the

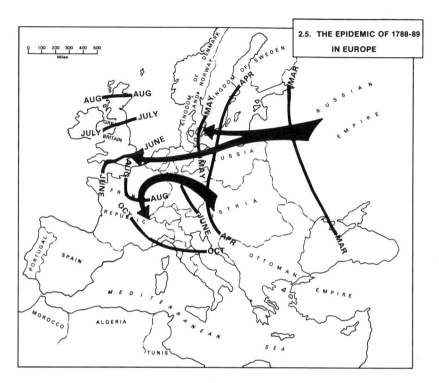

2.5. THE EPIDEMIC OF 1788-89 IN EUROPE

same month that the epidemic broke out in Paris,[97] and northern France (Lille, Douai) in September.[98] In October, the epidemic reached its maximum extent, with outbreaks in Geneva and in several cities in northern Italy.[99]

In America, influenza was widespread a year later, in the fall of 1789. The earliest reports were from Georgia[100] and New York City[101] in September. It also appeared in Norfolk, Virginia, in late September.[102] Philadelphia was infected at the end of the month, apparently by travelers from New York. The epidemic advanced northward from New York, reaching Hartford in mid-October,[103] Boston in early November, and Nova Scotia in December.[104] Influenza seems to have spread well into the interior; it was said to have attacked the "Indians in the wilderness,"[105] and there was a severe outbreak near the Niagara frontier.[106] The disease was also transmitted to the West Indies, with October epidemics in Jamaica,[107] Martinique, Eustasius, St. Kitts, and Dominica. Grenada was infected in November by shipping from islands farther north.[108] There are very vague indications that influenza was active in "Spanish South America" during the winter of 1789–1790.[109] Flu returned to the northeastern United States in the spring and fall of 1790 and again in the spring of 1791.

Many people contracted it more than once, suggesting that the original virus had undergone substantial drift.[110] The agent of the American epidemic was probably related to the 1788 virus in Europe; the scattered outbreaks in September 1789 suggest pre-seeding in several ports, but it is unclear why there was no epidemic for a year.

The epidemic of 1788–1789 was not especially severe in either Europe or North America. Morbidity was estimated at 50 percent in Munich,[111] and was said to be high in Warsaw,[112] Vienna,[113] Manchester,[114] Paris,[115] Norfolk, Virginia,[116] Philadelphia,[117] and the West Indies,[118] but no author reported much mortality. Those who died were almost always old and/or chronically ill. Quantitative information is almost nonexistent. In Westmoreland Parish, Jamaica, there were only thirteen or fourteen deaths out of a population of 5,500 slaves, 200 whites, and "many free persons of colour."[119] In contrast to 1782, weekly bills of mortality in England showed no increase.[120]

The pandemic status of the 1788–1789 epidemic is unclear. High morbidity, clear patterns of spread, and possible transatlantic transmission suggest that it might have been a true pandemic. It was, however, clearly much less spectacular than the 1781–1782 episode, and it received much less attention from contemporary observers. The 1788–1789 epidemic must remain classified as only a possible pandemic, although it seems more likely to have been a real pandemic than the epidemic of 1761–1762.

The three pandemics and two possible pandemics described in this chapter have many features in common. All spread from east to west in Europe and, when influenza apparently crossed the Atlantic to cause epidemics in 1732 and 1789, it took the virus a year to get established. Europeans, long accustomed to the notion that dangerous things like plague and Turks came out of the mysterious East, quickly adopted a xenogenic view of the origins of epidemic influenza. It came from the East, with Russia a prime suspect. The American epidemiologist Currie vividly expressed this view in 1792. Influenza, like smallpox and measles, came to America on ship from Europe, and Europe was infected from Asia or the "domains of the Despotic Turk."[121]

The evidence from Russia is very fragmentary, at least in the present state of research, but the pattern of east-west diffusion into Europe seems to have been established only in the eighteenth century.[122] While this could well be an artifact of our scanty knowledge of earlier centuries, political changes are probably relevant. Peter the Great's revolutionary foreign policy broke Russia's relative isolation and put the country into much closer political and economic relations with the West. He constructed a new capital at St. Petersburg and acquired Sweden's holdings on the eastern shore of the Baltic, including the major port of Riga, at the conclusion of the Great Northern War in 1721. These developments, which put Russia into direct contact with the West and increased the speed and volume of trade, obviously could have had epidemiological consequences. Several eighteenth- and early nineteenth-century epidemics have a definite Baltic flavor about them, although how much of this is due to a Russian factor, the extensive commerce in the Baltic, or the efficiency of disease reporting in the Kingdom of Prussia can be only conjectural.

The geographical progression of epidemic influenza was so obvious to eighteenth-century observers that even the most fervent anticontagionists had to deal with it. The fact that influenza frequently advanced against prevailing winds and seemed to radiate out from cities probably contributed to the rise of contagionist thought by the 1780s.

The five most important epidemics of the century each took several months to traverse Europe. There is no evidence that their pace changed over the century, which is hardly surprising given the absence of major innovations in transportation. Italy and the Iberian Peninsula were the last to be affected, and the maps suggest fairly rapid movement through northern Germany and a retarding effect in the Alps. Unfortunately, we usually cannot specify routes of spread in any detail, but it appears that influenza roughly followed major paths of commerce and tended to establish itself in cities before diffusing into the countryside.

Outside the tropics, influenza is frequently a disease of the cold months. This is clearly the case for the 1729–1730 and 1732–1733 pandemics and in North America in 1789. Yet there was substantial summertime influenza activity in 1762, 1782, and 1788. There is also evidence suggesting possible pre-seeding during the summer months, which led to fall outbreaks, in North America in 1732 and 1789 and in Europe in 1729. Observations of possible associations with diseases among animals will be discussed in the concluding chapter.

There was nothing surprising about the impact of influenza on public health in the eighteenth century. Morbidity reports, inevitably impressionistic, stress high attack rates with little or no discrimination as to age, sex, or socioeconomic status. Influenza caused temporary inconvenience and disruption of normal activities, but it rarely lasted more than four to six weeks in any given locality. Case-mortality rates were low, with most deaths occurring among the elderly or the chronically ill, and there were a few suggestions that pregnant women were especially vulnerable. The role of secondary pneumonias was clearly understood. There is no evidence that any of these epidemics produced anything at all resembling the high mortality and peculiar age-specific death rates observed in 1918.

On a virological level, there must have been at least three H/N shifts to account for the pandemics that began in 1729, 1732, and 1781. Two other shifts for the epidemics beginning in 1761 and 1788 are possible; 1788 seems more likely to have been a true pandemic. The repeated outbreaks in North America in 1789–1791 could be interpreted as evidence of viral draft. The only surprising thing about the number and timing of pandemics is the close proximity of those that started in 1729 and 1732. There is no substantial evidence on the geographical origins of pandemic strains, but somewhere in the Russian Empire seems at least plausible. Even though influenza was active in Japan in 1733 and 1781, there really is nothing to indicate Chinese origins except for extrapolations from the 1957, 1968, and 1977 pandemics and recent studies of viruses in domestic ducks in Hong Kong and southern China.

3
Epidemic and Pandemic Influenza
1799–1858

The general socioeconomic environment and the state of medical knowledge prevailing in the first half of the nineteenth century showed many continuities with the previous century, although changes were underway in both areas that would have major consequences for influenza in 1889 and after. For most of the period, despite the beginnings of the Industrial Revolution, improvements in transportation were incremental. Only by 1847 was the developing railroad system a factor in influenza diffusion. Urban growth continued, with cities like London and Paris absorbing ever-increasing numbers of rural migrants, but the majority of Europeans continued to live in villages and small towns.

The pace of medical advance began to quicken in the early decades of the century, especially with the rise of clinical studies and pathological anatomy in Paris.[1] But these developments, while crucial for the future rise of scientific medicine, had little immediate impact on the perception or treatment of influenza. Most medical observers in this period believed in some sort of miasmatic theory for the origin and spread of the disease; indeed, contagionists were less influential in the 1830s and 1840s than they had been in the 1780s or even in 1803.[2] The causes of influenza, whether meteorological phenomena, specific miasmatic poisons, or even perhaps direct person-to-person contagion, were hotly debated. One British writer even suggested that "animalcules" in the air caused influenza, measles, and smallpox—an early flirtation with a germ theory.[3] Another source of controversy was the possibility that influenza somehow heralded the cholera epidemic of 1831–1832 or was by unknown mechanisms transformed into cholera.[4]

Therapy remained essentially unchanged. Although some physicians inclined toward the more extensive bleedings and other depletions of the "heroic" approach popular in the early decades of the century, most remained cautious and tried to avoid further weakening the patient. Treatment was generally mild, symptomatic, and supportive in uncomplicated cases, with only the more therapeutically aggressive physicians employing drastic bleeding, and inducing sweating, purging, and vomiting in their sicker patients.[5]

One important trend in the 1830s and 1840s was the growing interest in vital statistics in several European countries. As the deleterious consequences of industrialization and urbanization for living conditions and public health became more evident, reformers pushed for censuses, surveys of conditions in cities and industries, and systematic collection of vital statistics to document problems and to try to find remedies.[6] Medical journals were by now much more numerous and the relevant medical literature much more abundant than in the eighteenth century. Both physicians and officials were more conscious of the value of numbers and rates for sickness and death from influenza and other diseases. Health statistics were, of course, still rudimentary. But although most of the data were collected in major cities and there were serious problems in assigning causes of death, much more can be learned about the public health impact of influenza than in earlier centuries.

In the nineteenth century, as in the eighteenth, there were at least three influenza pandemics and several other major epidemics. As in the 1700s, two of the nineteenth-century pandemics were clustered early in the fourth decade (1830–1831 and 1833) and one, the most spectacular, developed late in the century (1889–1890). Lesser outbreaks, sometimes connected and sometimes contemporaneous but independent of each other, took place in 1799–1800, 1802–1803, 1805–1807, 1825–1827, 1850–1851, and 1857–1858.

Influenza was very active in the early years of the Napoleonic wars, especially between 1799 and 1807. The diffusion and impact of the disease were almost certainly facilitated by troop movements and wartime dislocations. For example, at various times Russian, Austrian, and Prussian armies operated over much of western Europe, English armies appeared on the Continent, and French forces ranged widely in Italy and central Europe.

The first epidemic of the century actually began in late 1799 in Russia, but it is best treated as a nineteenth-century episode.[7] Flu was reported in Moscow in October 1799 and apparently spread north and east in November to Vologda, Archangel, and Kazan. In December, the Baltic region, including St. Petersburg, Riga, and Mittau, was attacked, and influenza advanced southwestward into the Ukraine, Podolia, and Volynia. Vilna in Lithuania, Lemberg (Lvov) in Austrian Galicia, and Krakow were attacked in January 1800, Warsaw and Prussia (including Königsberg) in February, and Vienna and Posen (Poznan) in April. The last gasps of the epidemic occurred in Saxony in April and Copenhagen in May (see Map 3.1).

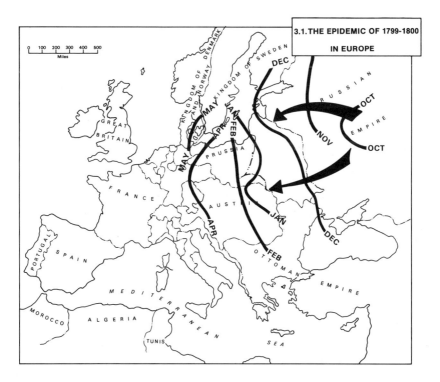

This outbreak was consistently described as mild. Although there was a clear pattern of east-west diffusion, this strain did not reach western Europe except along the Baltic, and southern Europe was totally unaffected. Scattered flu outbreaks in central and western Germany in the fall of 1800 may have been late consequences of this episode. It was not, in any case, a true pandemic.

The signing of the Peace of Amiens in March 1802 provided a temporary break in the wars, but it may have been a stimulus for the influenza epidemic that swept western Europe in 1802–1803.[8] Possibly the virus reached France with veterans returning home from the battlefields, and/or recombination/mutation took place in the barracks. The epidemic began in Paris in September 1802. Influenza was reported in Aachen in October and was widespread in France during November and December. The disease reached Milan and parts of the northern Rhineland in January 1803. England and Ireland were attacked in the same month, with earliest reports from the port cities of London, Newcastle, Liverpool, and Dublin. Influenza diffused over Britain from these foci during February and March[9] and spread over western Germany during the same months. It was active in Geneva and northern Italy in March. This epidemic, which clearly radiated outward from France, was restricted to western Europe. Contemporary reports stressed high morbidity and low mortality.[10] Enough deaths occurred, however, especially among the elderly, for one observer to remind his readers of numerous deaths in London and Paris and admonish them that this is therefore "no trivial matter."[11] Despite Beveridge's assertion, based on presumably unrelated reports of influenza in China and Brazil (Rio de Janeiro) in 1801, this epidemic cannot be directly linked to events of 1799–1800, and cannot be considered a pandemic.[12]

Two other periods of influenza activity prior to the century's first pandemic deserve brief mention.[13] Scattered and perhaps unrelated foci were active in the West Indies in late 1805, in various areas of Europe in 1806, and in the United States in 1807. In New York, the epidemic apparently began in New York City in early summer and spread over the rest of the state by late August. Morbidity was high, but there were few deaths.[14] The disease was again widely reported in the United States in late 1825 and early 1826, in Mexico in May, in Peru in September 1826, and in western Siberia in early 1827. The Siberian epidemic, at least, must have been independent.

The first pandemic of the century took place in 1830–1831. Influenza epidemics occurred in four widely separated regions during these years: China and Southeast Asia, India, Europe, and North America. In Europe, the epidemic spread westward from Russia in a style that had become familiar in the eighteenth century. North America was almost certainly infected from Europe and India may have been also. There is no documented connection between the Southeast Asian and European outbreaks, but it is possible that influenza developed in China and spread to the Philippines and Indonesia by sea trade, and traveled across Siberia to European Russia.

The origins of this pandemic are unclear, although there are vague references to influenza in Canton in October and November 1829.[15] This is especially interesting in light of recent speculation on South China as a birthplace for pandemic strains. There are further notices of influenza in undefined areas of China in January and September 1830.[16] The January episode was apparently coastal, as the crew of a British ship was struck on the 25th "at China."[17] Manila suffered severely beginning in early September. It is quite likely that ships from China introduced the disease to the Philippines; later in the same month, on the 18th, a British ship coming from China did reach Manila with active cases.[18]

Influenza presumably spread southward in the Philippines during the fall months (Map 3.2). By January 1831 the disease had reached

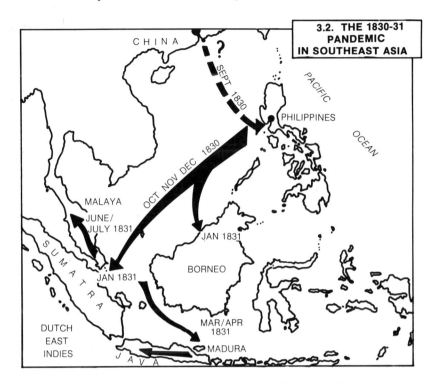

Borneo and Sumatra in the Dutch East Indies.[19] In late March a
serious epidemic began at Grisee, in Surabaya Province, northeast
Java. It prevailed in the interior of Surabaya and in the nearby island
of Madura in mid-April, and began to advance slowly westward,
reaching the western end of Java by early June.[20] Continuing its
advance in a northwesterly direction, flu broke out in Singapore in
mid-June, Malacca at the end of the month, and in Penang in the
middle of July.[21] There are no further data on the pandemic in Asia,
except for two localities in India in 1832 to be discussed later, and
the fact that Japan experienced an epidemic in 1831–1832.[22]

In Europe, Moscow was attacked in November 1830 and St.
Petersburg in January 1831 (Map 3.3).[23] The origins of the pandemic
in Europe are unknown, but it is tempting to postulate that a new
virus spread from China through the Russian outposts in Siberia and
across the Urals, or else crossed Sinkiang to the independent Moslem states of modern Soviet Central Asia. Either route would have
required transmission over thousands of miles of sparsely populated
territory. At any rate, influenza advanced to the Baltic region at
Mittau and Dorpat (Tartu) in February and to Warsaw in March.
Breslau (Wroclaw), Berlin,[24] and East Prussia were afflicted in April,

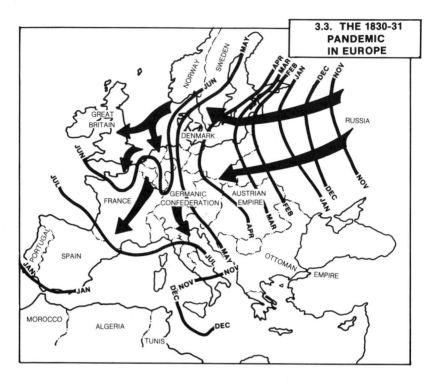

3.3. THE 1830-31
PANDEMIC
IN EUROPE

and flu reached Budapest, Prague, Vienna, Hamburg, central Germany, Denmark,[25] Finland, and Sweden in May. Influenza prevailed in June in western Germany, England,[26] Scotland,[27] Paris,[28] and northern France, the same month that it visited Singapore. Extension to the Low Countries, southern France, and Geneva[29] took place in July, and after a summer lull, influenza advanced southward to Rome in mid-November,[30] to Naples and to Sicily in December, and to Spain and Gibraltar in January 1832. The east-west progression of the epidemic is evident in the reports from Prussian military bases shown in Table 3.1.

Information on the epidemic in the United States is meager, but it was almost certainly introduced by ships from Europe. The mid-Atlantic region was the first focus, with initial reports from Philadelphia and New Jersey. Peaks were reported in Philadelphia and Boston in the week of 10–17 December 1831,[31] and Cincinnati may have had its first cases as early as mid-November.[32] Influenza spread southward along the Atlantic Coast,[33] reaching rural Burke County, Georgia, in February 1832.[34] By this time, the disease had covered "nearly the entire United States,"[35] from the Atlantic Coast to the Mississippi.

Table 3.1   The Spread of Influenza in Prussian Garrisons, 1831

Region	Place	Date of first appearance
East Prussia	Memel	4 March
East Prussia	Tilsit	13 March
East Prussia	Insterburg	13 March
East Prussia	Königsberg	17 March
Silesia	Gleiwitz	23 March
Silesia	Posen	25 March
Central Germany	Magdeburg	8 April
Central Germany	Erfurt	20 April
Western Germany	Minden	1 May
Western Germany	Mainz	15 May
Western Germany	Cologne	Beginning
Western Germany	Koblenz	of
Western Germany	Aix-la-Chapelle	June
Luxemburg	Luxemburg	10 June

Source: O. Leichtenstern. "Influenza," in *Malaria, Influenza, and Dengue*, ed. Julius Mannaberg and O. Leichtenstern (English trans. Philadelphia, 1905), 537.

As noted earlier, there was flu in India in April 1832. The only reports are of sharp outbreaks in two interior cities, Indore[36] and Merut[37] (north of Delhi), but the epidemic must have been much more widespread. There was another, perhaps related outbreak in Bangalore in December 1832.[38] There may be a connection with the Indonesian-Malayan events of March–July 1831, but the introduction of influenza via shipping from Europe seems more plausible. Two other hypotheses deserve mention. The Indian epidemic(s) could have been local and independent or, just possibly, India could have been the birthplace of the 1833 pandemic.

Although quantitative data are rare, observers consistently reported high morbidity and low case-mortality. In Manila and at Penang, so many people were sick that normal social and commercial activities were disrupted, but few died.[39] In Buitenborg Province, Java, Dutch officials reported 51,588 cases with 277 deaths in a population of 219,415. The morbidity rate (23.5 percent) is probably low because of underreporting, but the mortality rate (1.3 percent) is not implausible. Surabaya Province (population 311,192) reported 15.5 percent morbidity and 0.3 percent mortality.[40] In Europe, the disease was considered widespread but mild.[41] Morbidity was estimated at only about 10 percent in Geneva,[42] but three-quarters of the population of Naples contracted influenza.[43] England had little mortality, and influenza had almost no impact on the London death returns,[44] but one observer estimated overall mortality in Glasgow at 2 percent.[45] In Boston, Massachusetts, total deaths were about 20 percent above normal; perhaps half of this was due to influenza and its complications.[46] Persons of all ages were susceptible,[47] but most fatal cases were among the elderly.

The 1830–1831 influenza spread rapidly, causing much morbidity but little mortality. In Europe, the United States, and Southeast Asia, at least, it behaved like a true pandemic. Relationships, if any, between the simultaneous outbreaks in Europe and Asia in the first half of 1831 are not clear. Given the early, albeit vague, reports from China, and the likelihood of maritime spread from China to Manila, the most economical hypothesis is that a new pandemic strain arose in China in 1829 or early 1830. It spread by sea to the Philippines, and either from there or directly from China to Indonesia and thence to Malaya. Meanwhile, it somehow spread across the Eurasian landmass, first appearing in the written record in Moscow, and going on through Europe and across the North Atlantic, and perhaps to India. Research with Chinese and Russian sources, especially in Siberian archives, might support or weaken this hypothesis. In any case, there was undoubtedly a true pandemic in 1830–1831.

Influenza was very quiet in 1832, but in 1833 a great epidemic, much more lethal than its predecessor, swept Europe from east to west. Turkey, Syria, and Egypt were also affected, but the epidemic did not reach the Western Hemisphere,[48] and, unless the 1831–1832 Japanese outbreak or the 1832 events in India are somehow related, most of Asia apparently was not attacked.

The path carved by the 1833 influenza epidemic was quite similar to that of the outbreak only two years earlier (Map 3.4). This is very unusual, but not unprecedented, since, as described in chapter 2, a similar pair of pandemics swept Europe in 1729–1730 and 1732–1733. Although some writers have treated 1831 and 1833 as part of the same epidemic,[49] this is a minority position; the episodes, as will be shown, were quite distinct.

Influenza was reported in January in Russian cities from Perm in the Urals to St. Petersburg on the Baltic.[50] Obviously, the disease must have prevailed in late 1832 over at least part of this vast area. In February influenza moved southeastward to Riga,[51] Reval (Tallinn), Memel, eastern Galicia (Brody), and Odessa, with invasion of East Prussia,[52] Poland, and Bohemia in the next month. By the end of March, influenza had also reached Helsingor (Denmark), Berlin, and Constantinople. Hungary, Vienna, and eastern Austria, Saxony, Denmark,[53] England,[54] Ireland, and Scotland were attacked in April, along with Paris and Bordeaux. Western Germany was bypassed until May, when it was struck, along with Stockholm,[55] western Austria, and parts of northern Italy and eastern Yugoslavia. Also in

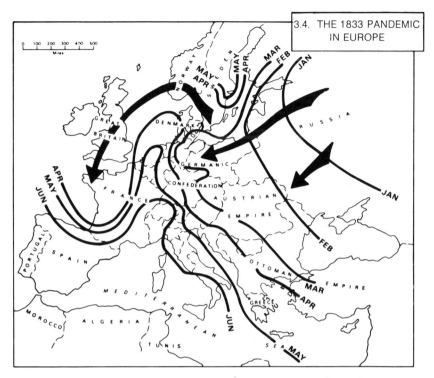

3.4. THE 1833 PANDEMIC IN EUROPE

May, the epidemic spread, probably from Constantinople, to Smyrna (Izmir), Syria, and Egypt (Cairo, Alexandria). In June flu finally reached the Low Countries, moved north in Sweden to Uppsala, and continued to spread in northern Italy.[56] As in 1831, Switzerland was also attacked late (September),[57] as were Naples[58] and Sicily (November). The epidemic apparently did not reach Spain or Portugal.

Morbidity was very high in most of Europe in 1833, apparently higher than in 1831. Tens of thousands fell ill in St. Petersburg and Berlin. Observers claimed that four-fifths of Memel's 10,000 people, one-third of the population of Königsberg (Kaliningrad)[59] and one-quarter of Stockholm's[60] inhabitants contracted influenza. Morbidity was estimated at 50 percent in Edinburgh,[61] and both London and Paris were said to equal Memel's 80 percent.[62] London's theaters shut down for lack of healthy actors, and the operations of the city police and the Bank of England were severely curtailed.[63] In Austria, one-half to one-third fell ill, in Bohemia two-thirds, but only one-sixth in Zurich.[64] Men and women, young and old, were all equally likely to be stricken.[65]

Mortality was also higher than in 1831 in the eyes of most contemporaries, although case-mortality rates remained low.[66] Death or burial records are available for a few cities. These data are too crude to estimate total or age-specific mortality, but total deaths did jump during the epidemic in Breslau, Vienna, Copenhagen,[67] Prague, Königsberg,[68] and Edinburgh.[69] As shown in Figure 3.1, flu caused heavy mortality in London from mid-April to mid-May, when the city had several thousand more deaths than normal. Birmingham was also hard hit.[70] For England as a whole, deaths in February 1833 were almost twice the normal toll for February.[71] Virtually all writers thought that the elderly and those with preexisting respiratory disease were most vulnerable.[72]

Epidemic influenza was much more restricted geographically in 1833 than in 1831, but it caused more morbidity and mortality in Europe. In this regard, it behaved like a second wave of a modern pandemic, which, as in 1890 and the fall of 1918, can be more lethal than the first wave.[73] Nonetheless, a whole year had passed without significant activity after 1831, and there is no hint in the literature that people who had contracted influenza in 1831 had gained any immunity against the 1833 virus. Both of these facts strongly suggest that two distinct viral types were involved. As in 1729–1730 and 1732–1733, Europe was swept by two classic east-west pandemics in close succession.

There was little further influenza activity in Europe until 1836–1837, when a severe epidemic engulfed the Continent. As in the case

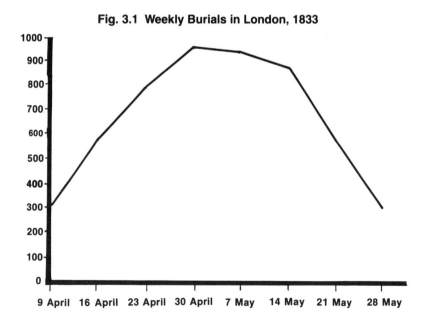

Fig. 3.1 Weekly Burials in London, 1833

of the previous epidemics, the origins of the 1836–1837 outbreak are
unclear, but in contrast, the pattern of spread was north to south,
rather than east to west (Map 3.5).

The earliest reports were from the Southern Hemisphere. In mid-
October 1836 flu was reportedly spreading in Sydney, Australia,[74]
and in the same month an epidemic developed in Cape Town, South
Africa.[75] Java and Penang were struck in November,[76] and flu was
recorded in the fall of 1836 in the Hudson's Bay Company's domains
in Northern Canada.[77] With this doubtful exception, influenza did
not reach the Western Hemisphere. The relationship, if any, of these
outbreaks to events in Europe is not known.

In Europe, the earliest reports were again from Russia. St. Petersburg was struck in November 1836, while influenza was still active
in Cape Town.[78] In December, flu struck London, Aberdeen, Stockholm, Copenhagen, and much of Denmark,[79] Berlin, Hamburg, and
two German Baltic ports, Lubeck and Greifswald. Indeed, the Baltic
region seems to have been an important early focus, and one influential writer believed that the epidemic started in Sweden and Denmark.[80] By the end of January influenza had reached Umeå in
northern Sweden,[81] had enveloped most of England and Ireland, and
had advanced generally southward, embracing most of Germany, the

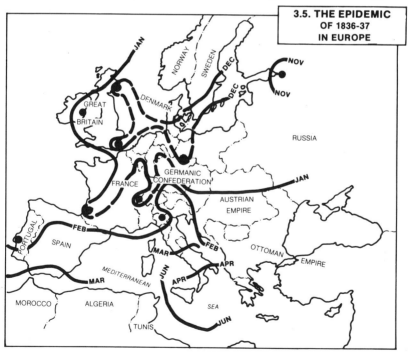

3.5. THE EPIDEMIC
OF 1836-37
IN EUROPE

Low Countries, Vienna, Paris, and even Bordeaux. Geneva was hit at the end of the month.[82] Outbreaks also began in January in Syria and Egypt. France and northern Italy were overrun in February, and flu swept the Rhineland and northern Spain. Lisbon was infected in early February by ships from England.[83] Again, most of Switzerland was attacked late, in March, and the epidemic reached Rome, Madrid, and Barcelona in the same month. Naples was not struck until May, Palermo[84] and Malta[85] in June. This epidemic did reach Iceland.[86] Thus, although the picture is far from clear, a general pattern of diffusion from northern Russia followed by a fairly rapid southward thrust from early foci in England and the Baltic is evident, with southern Italy and the Iberian Peninsula, as usual, being involved last. Pétrequin and Lombard noted that big cities in any given region of France, England, Italy, or Switzerland were attacked first, with subsequent radiation outward to small towns and then the countryside.[87]

The geographical pattern is more complex than for the previous epidemics, however, raising the possibility of pre-seeding of virus during the summer and fall of 1836. The 1836–1837 virus was too late to have been a "second wave" of the 1833 pandemic, but it could have been a variant of the 1833 strain that had drifted enough to evade host immunity, spread quietly during the fall, and exploded when cold weather created favorable conditions. Another possibility is that the outbreaks reported from Australia, South Africa, and Southeast Asia are the only recorded traces of a pandemic that swept the Southern Hemisphere in the middle of 1836. The virus could have reached Europe by fall, spread quietly, and caused a series of outbreaks when winter came. A similar pattern took place in 1957 and 1968. Early involvement of Britain by colonial trade is understandable, but events in the Baltic region are more difficult to explain with this hypothesis.

The most plausible scenario remains an early involvement of Russia, with subsequent extension to the Baltic and then quick movement along trade routes to Britain. The fact that England was attacked so soon would shift diffusion patterns somewhat, with north-south movement more evident than the east-west component. Neither of the pre-seeding arguments can, however, be dismissed on the existing evidence. In any case, this was probably a new pandemic strain, the third in less than a decade, and it was the most severe influenza to strike Europe since 1782.

Extensive morbidity was widely reported. A British doctor wrote of an "immense number of victims."[88] More than half the population of Geneva[89] and Copenhagen fell ill, and almost every household was affected in Stockholm.[90] Another observer in Geneva estimated mortality in that city at slightly under 50 percent.[91] A similar figure was reported for Paris and Lyon, and close to 75 percent contracted flu in Florence.[92] And, as in 1833, there was no evidence that exposure to prior epidemics conveyed any immunity to the new strain.[93]

While case-mortality rates remained low, total mortality was extensive, and the epidemic was almost universally described as more deadly than the two previous pandemics. In Dublin, flu claimed about 3,000 lives, more than the 1832 cholera epidemic, and the disease was much more severe than in 1833.[94] Total deaths doubled during the epidemic in one Paris *arrondissement*[95] and were elevated in the city as a whole,[96] and unusually high death tolls were recorded in such cities as London,[97] Berlin, Hannover,[98] Stockholm,[99] Geneva,[100] and Glasgow.[101] A contemporary survey of British doctors suggested an overall case-fatality rate of 2.0 to 2.5 percent.[102] Most of the deaths were among the elderly and the chronically ill and were associated with secondary pneumonias.[103] A London doctor captured the tone of the literature well. "We have been visited by one of the most direful scourges, in the form of influenza, that has occurred within the memory of the oldest practitioner, and which in its consequences will be found to have been far more fatal than the cholera."[104]

Better quantitative data, even though scattered and expressed as total excess deaths rather than cause-specific mortality, are available for 1837 than for any previous influenza epidemic. Comparisons of monthly deaths in 1837 with the tolls for two previous years in three French cities are shown in Table 3.2. The tenth *arrondissement* of Paris experienced a doubling of deaths in February 1837; Lyon's

Table 3.2   Mortality in Three French Cities, 1835–1837

	Paris[a] (10th *Arrondissement*)			Lyon[b]			Limoges[c]		
	1835	1836	1837	1835	1836	1837	1835	1836	1837
January	309	293	301	—	—	—	111	95	102
February	125	138	286	428	410	640	104	102	114
March	—	—	—	487	426	666	111	113	188

[a]"Note pour servir à l'histoire de la grippe de Paris," *Gazette médicale de Paris*, 2d ser., 5 (1837): 143.
[b]M. Pétriquin. "Recherches pour servir à l'histoire générale de la grippe de 1837 en France et en Italie," *Gazette médicale de Paris*, 2d ser., 5 (1837): 808.
[c]1–15 February only.

total was far above normal in February and March; and deaths did not rise in the smaller, more southerly city of Limoges until March. London recorded a sharp rise in total deaths and in those ascribed to influenza in late January (Table 3.3). Death peaks occurred, as usual, about four weeks after the onset of the epidemic. Age-specific rates were not published, but even the absolute numbers of deaths by age in London show heavy mortality among the elderly (Fig. 3.2).

The most detailed reports came from Denmark. Influenza became epidemic in December 1836, and the peak in excess mortality predictably occurred in January (Table 3.4). Figures for deaths by four broad age groups, shown in Table 3.5, confirm that most of the excess mortality was in persons over 50, and there was no significant increase in those under 25. In Denmark, as must have been true in most countries, there was considerable geographical variation in mortality. Table 3.6 shows that the four island provinces (Copenhagen, Sjelland, Fyn, and Lolland-Falster) were hit earlier and generally less severely than the Jutland provinces (Alborg, Viborg, Aarhuus, and Ribe). It is possible, even likely, that comparable unpublished mortality data exist for countries like England, Sweden, and Prussia, and the Danish reports serve to provide useful illustrations of some general trends in mortality.

There was scattered influenza activity in Germany, Austria, and Hungary in the early months of 1841; in Belgium, England, and France in early 1842; in the United States during the summer of 1843; and portions of western Germany and Switzerland in early

---

Table 3.3   Total and Influenza Mortality in London, 1837

Week ending	Total burials	Influenza deaths
3 January	228	0
10 January	284	0
17 January	477	13
24 January	871	106
31 January	860	99
7 February	598	63
14 February	558	35
21 February	350	20
28 February	321	8
7 March	262	4
Total	4,809	348

Source: Heberden, "On the Late Influenza," *London Medical Gazette*, 20 (1837): 51; Great Britain, *Annual Report of the Registrar General of Births, Deaths, and Marriages in England* 10 (1847), xlii.

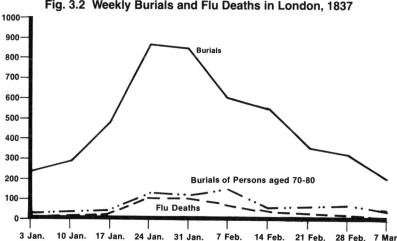

Fig. 3.2 Weekly Burials and Flu Deaths in London, 1837

1844. Yet nothing resembling a major epidemic developed until 1847.

The epidemic of 1847–1848, considered a true pandemic by many authors, primarily affected western Europe and the Mediterranean (Map 3.6). East and South Asia were not involved, nor were the Americas, with the possible exception of a minor late outbreak in the West Indies in October and November 1848.[105] Hirsch's listing of a related epidemic in Hawaii in January 1848[106] seems very weakly supported by the original source[107] and must be discounted.

As in the three epidemics already discussed, there was a possible precursor with unknown connections with the main epidemic.[108] The early activity was in Russia, where Moscow and nearby Yaroslavl had flu in January and February. A violent outbreak struck

Table 3.4   Excess Mortality in Denmark, December 1836–May 1837

Month	Deaths 1836–37	Average deaths 1835, '36, '38, '39	Excess in 1837
December 1836	2,285	2,327	−42
January 1837	3,589	2,761	828
February	3,063	2,635	428
March	3,139	2,994	145
April	3,221	2,978	243
May	2,872	2,907	−35

Source: A. F. Bremer, and E. Fenger, "Om Influenza-Epidemierne i Danmark i Aarene 1825 til 1844," *Det Kongelige Medicinske Selskabs i København Skrifter* (1848), 226–27.

Table 3.5   Excess Mortality in Denmark by Age Group, 1837 (stillbirths excluded)

	Under 11 Years		11-25		26-50		Over 50	
	1837	Average 1835, '36, '38, '39	1837	Average 1835, '36, '38, '39	1837	Average 1835, '36, '38, '39	1837	Average 1835, '36, '38, '39
January	1,088	1,039	214	206	486	405	1,610	942
February	924	1,005	189	192	443	385	1,362	898
March	1,110	1,128	222	230	481	424	1,155	1,034
April	1,058	1,125	267	243	504	466	1,237	984
Total	4,180	4,297	892	871	1,914	1,680	5,364	3,858

Source: A. F. Bremer and E. Fenger, "Om Influenza-Epidemierne i Danmark i Aarene 1825 til 1844," *Det Kongelige Medicinske Selskabs i København Skrifter*, (1848), 228.

Table 3.6   Excess Mortality in Denmark, 1837, by Province

Province		January	February	March	April	Total
Copenhagen	Excess deaths[a]	64	-87	45	46	68
	Percent excess	20	-29	15	15	6
Sjelland	Excess deaths[a]	227	-30	-88	-56	53
	Percent excess	30	-4	-10	-6	2
Fyn	Excess deaths[a]	203	43	54	100	400
	Percent excess	64	14	16	29	30
Lolland-	Excess deaths[a]	-6	-8	-37	-40	-91
Falster	Percent excess	-3	-5	-21	-22	-13
Alborg	Excess deaths[a]	167	70	13	13	263
	Percent excess	66	27	5	5	25
Viborg	Excess deaths[a]	65	100	42	54	261
	Percent excess	33	57	22	29	35
Aarhuus	Excess deaths[a]	47	151	2	34	234
	Percent excess	11	36	0	8	13
Ribe	Excess deaths[a]	62	189	115	92	458
	Percent excess	21	61	33	26	35

[a]Compared to monthly averages for 1835, 1836, 1838, and 1839.

Source: A. F. Bremer and E. Fenger, "Om Influenza-Epidemierne i Danmark i Aarene 1825 til 1844," *Det Kongelige Medicinske Selskabs i København Skrifter* (1848), 230.

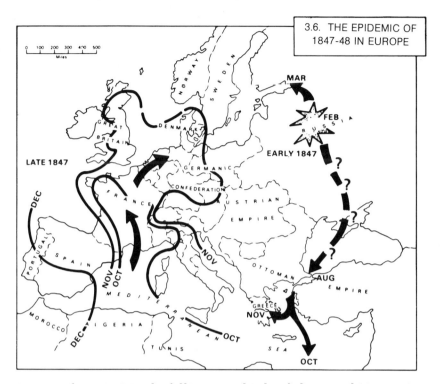

3.6. THE EPIDEMIC OF 1847-48 IN EUROPE

St. Petersburg in March, felling two-thirds of the population.[109] In sharp constrast to past epidemics, the disease did not spread westward and, unless it moved southward to Turkey during the spring and summer, the Russian epidemic seems to have remained strictly local.

The first definite appearance of what became a major epidemic was in Constantinople in late August.[110] In October, Alexandria (Egypt) was infected, and Malta's epidemic began in the middle of the month. Southern France was also attacked in October, probably early in the month. Lyon was swiftly engulfed; by the end of October, Nice, the northwestern coast of Italy, and even Rennes in Brittany were beginning to report cases.[111] In November the disease advanced rapidly over France and Britain, the Low Countries, northern Germany, Denmark,[112] and Bohemia. It reached Athens in the middle of the month, probably directly from Turkey.[113] During December there was further spread in Britain and western Germany, and there were outbreaks in Algiers and Geneva.[114] In Spain, Madrid[115] and Barcelona[116] were struck in the last days of the year. Liège, Naples,[117] and Munich did not get influenza until January 1848, and Berne,[118] protected by the Alps, was not affected until mid-February. It is surprising that the epidemic seems to have died out then, even though it was the prime season, winter. Influenza lingered in Denmark through January, but died out before the spring shipping season opened, so Iceland was not infected.[119]

The geography of the 1847–1848 epidemic was peculiar. Sweden, normally an early target, escaped completely,[120] and the epidemic remained confined to western and southern Europe and North Africa.[121] There was no further involvement of Russia, and eastern Europe was not touched. It was a Mediterranean epidemic, like that of 1580, with a rapid penetration of France, and subsequent radiation in a manner reminiscent of 1803.[122] Newly developing but still segmented railroad systems probably facilitated spread in northern France, Belgium, and northern Germany.

Morbidity in 1847–1848 was extensive, but perhaps less than in the previous epidemics. One Londoner in four got flu;[123] the proportion was one in three in Geneva,[124] and guessed at one in two in Paris.[125] The disease was generally mild,[126] except in Geneva, where there was a heavy toll, particularly among the elderly,[127] and in Belgium.[128] In London, there were over 5,000 more deaths than normal during the epidemic period, mostly among the aged. Table 3.7 shows the sharp mortality peak in early December. Some London districts had twice the death rates of healthier ones, and rural areas had lower mortality rates than the capital.[129] For all of England and Wales, influenza was registered as the cause of 12,844 deaths in 1847–1848, a figure that did not include deaths attributed to pneumonia and other respiratory diseases.[130]

Table 3.7   Total Mortality and Influenza Mortality in London, 1847

Week ending	Total deaths	Influenza deaths
30 October	945	1
6 November	1,052	2
13 November	1,098	4
20 November	1,086	4
27 November	1,677	36
4 December	2,454	198
11 December	2,416	374
18 December	1,946	270
25 December	1,247	142
1 January	1,599	127
Total	15,520	1,158

Source: Great Britain, *Annual Report of the Registrar General of Births, Deaths, and Marriages in England* 10 (1847), xxvii–xxix.

The 1847–1848 epidemic is puzzling. It was widespread and severe enough to attract a great deal of attention, but it did not seem infectious enough to diffuse as widely as in the 1830s. The apparent disappearance of the disease in mid-winter is quite unusual. In sum, the common assertion[131] that 1847–1848 was a pandemic year now seems unjustified. A fairly substantial epidemic in its own right, its promotion to pandemic status is probably the result of its occurrence in the center of medical writing, western Europe.

In December 1850, influenza was reported in the West Indies and along the Pacific coast of South America in Peru and Chile. An outbreak in Germany from January to March 1851 was almost certainly unrelated. Again, in 1857 influenza was widespread in the Western Hemisphere. Flu was present in Panama in August and the West Indies and the Peruvian and Chilean coasts in September, with an isolated report from Vancouver Island, British Columbia, in the same month. In December, there were simultaneous reports from much of Europe, including Russia, Germany, Bohemia, Belgium, and France. Italy was attacked in January 1858, and Athens in February.[132] Yet despite the assertions of Beveridge,[133] there are no apparent linkages between what seem to have been at least two distinct foci; and the 1857–1858 influenza cannot be considered a pandemic.

After the late 1850s, influenza was relatively quiet for many years. There were localized outbreaks from time to time, but nothing resembling a major epidemic. As the dramatic events of the 1830s and 1840s receded into the past, epidemic influenza became an almost forgotten disease. In 1889, when the next great pandemic swept the world, most doctors initially felt that they were confronted with something quite new.

The 1830–1848 period was remarkable for widespread influenza activity. There had been no definite pandemic since 1782. Pandemics occurred in 1830–1831 and 1833, and there was a probable pandemic in 1836–1837 and a serious but nonpandemic episode in 1847–48. The first two, and probably the third as well, spread in what Pyle and Patterson have characterized as a massive frontal movement pattern. The 1847–1848 epidemic seems to fit a multiple-sequential pattern, with epicenters in Turkey, southern France, and possibly Russia.[134] As in 1729 and 1730, influenza A virus "shifted" repeatedly in the span of a few years, and, as in the eighteenth century, there was roughly a half-century between a flurry of viral change and the next pandemic.

The geographical origins of these pandemics remain unknown. China may have given birth to the 1830–1831 pandemic, but this cannot be proven. Early reports from Russia, in the eighteenth and, nineteenth centuries, are at least as likely to reflect cultural assumptions and the limits of medical writers' knowledge as the actual geographical origins of pandemics. It is possible that Chinese and Russian archives contain information that would help to resolve these problems.

The 1830–1831 and 1833 pandemics, and perhaps 1836–1837 as well, followed the general pattern set by the three eighteenth-century pandemics, with the first European reports (but not necessarily the ultimate origins) from central Russia. Diffusions took place westward through Europe, with late involvement of Switzerland and especially Spain and southern Italy. Indeed, the most distant areas were reached more quickly in the eighteenth century, as there was a summer halt in both 1830 and 1833. Except for this, rates of spread were quite similar in all five pandemics—not surprising in view of the limited improvements in transportation facilities in most of Europe. Somewhat more rapid movement is suggested in 1836–1837 and 1847–1848. The former could represent pre-seeding, although the pace of the epidemic did not exceed travel rates. Only by 1847–1848 were there embryonic rail lines to assist the diffusion of the virus.

All four outbreaks considered here showed high morbidity and low case-mortality. In any given city, influenza flourished for about four to six weeks, causing temporary but soon-forgotten disruption of daily life. Although mortality was not comparable to that experienced in the fall of 1918, total deaths were high, often higher than during the terrifying cholera pandemic of 1831–1832, because so many people did get sick. As is usual in flu epidemics, most deaths were among the elderly. High mortality among young adults was peculiar to the pandemic of 1918–1919.

4

Pandemic Influenza
1889–1901

The great pandemic of 1889–1890, the first to occur in modern times, is far better documented than any of its predecessors. It is the first influenza epidemic that can be demonstrated to have been truly global in scope and the first for which the public health impact can be described in any detail. The behavior of this pandemic resembles twentieth-century pandemics far more closely than it does those of earlier times.

Europe and parts of North America had experienced major socio-economic changes since mid-century. Urbanization and industrialization had reached much higher levels in Britain and western Europe, and were spreading rapidly to the southern and eastern portions of the Continent and to parts of North America. Revolutionary developments in transportation allowed influenza to move from city to city and into the countryside at unprecedented speeds. Better roads and canals played a role, but the crucial innovation was the railroad network that now covered Europe from the Urals to London and Lisbon, and extended from coast to coast in North America. Equally important for transmission to port cities and between continents was the enormous increase in the volume and speed of maritime commerce associated with modern steamships. Growing long-distance trade and late-nineteenth-century imperialism were forging much stronger links between Europe and the Americas, Africa, Asia, and the Pacific than had ever existed before. The rapid global diffusion of influenza provides a graphic illustration of how the world was becoming a single interconnecting entity.

In most of Europe, and in a few other places that tried to keep up with Europe's models, governments had created active agencies to monitor and improve health conditions. Census taking and compilation of vital statistics were considered essential activities for modern European governments or for those, like Egypt, many of the states of the United States, and some of the Latin American republics, who were striving to emulate European standards. Data from urban areas were still usually more complete and accurate than returns from the countryside, but several western European countries and other places, including a few American states, provided good coverage of their entire territories. In the aftermath of the epidemic, England, Germany, Switzerland, Sweden, and some other countries published detailed studies of their experiences with influenza. These valuable official documents will be cited repeatedly in this chapter. Such documentation was almost unknown for earlier influenza epidemics,[1] when the few collective investigations were conducted by medical societies who depended on responses to questionnaires by physicians interested enough to fill them out. This type of study, which could of course provide much useful information, was still employed by private and official groups in several places and supplemented governmental efforts.[2]

The medical establishment and the state of medical knowledge were also much more "modern" in 1889 than they had been a half-century earlier. The number and professionalism of doctors and their journals had grown enormously. As medicine absorbed the insights and values of the burgeoning natural sciences, a much more critical and quantitative atmosphere began to pervade the literature. Humoral remedies like bleeding and purging were discredited; influenza therapy was now symptomatic and supportive. The triumph of the germ theory, so ably developed by Pasteur, Koch, and their followers, had revolutionized thinking about the cause of influenza. It had become difficult to consider influenza as anything but a discrete entity with a discrete cause; it probably could not change into or develop from cholera or any other epidemic disease. The germ theory had led to a substantial decline of miasmatic theories among leading medical writers, although older ideas were still common among practitioners.[3] The rapid transmission of influenza along communications routes convinced most authorities that influenza was contagious and must be caused by a microorganism.[4] Many investigators tried to isolate an agent, and one microbe described during this pandemic, Pheiffer's bacillus, remained a prime suspect until after 1918. In sum, doctors and public health officials, convinced of the importance of precise observations, quantification, and scientific standards, and thinking in terms of a specific disease transmitted from person to person, operated in an intellectual environment that generated much more abundant and useful data on epidemic influenza than had ever appeared before. For the first time, maps were used to illustrate the spread of the disease,[5] and elaborate statistical tables measured, however imperfectly, its impact on the population.

The pandemic of 1889 came as a total surprise. There had been no major epidemic since 1847–1848, and it took some intellectual effort and study of works like Hirsch's treatise and older contemporary accounts to recognize that the disease then sweeping the world was the same one that a few elderly physicians remembered from a half-century earlier. There had, of course, been scattered outbreaks in the intervening decades, and there was retrospective interest in local epidemics in the later 1880s that might have been predecessors of the great pandemic. For example, influenza was active in New Caledonia, California, France, and Zurich in 1863–1864, in the first three months of 1873 in the United States, and in the United States, France, Germany, Australia, and Sweden in 1873–1874. Indeed, Hirsch thought that there was a true pandemic in 1873–1874.[6]

Russia saw considerable influenza activity in the late 1880s. Local outbreaks developed in St. Petersburg every winter from 1885 through 1888,[7] and most provinces reported at least a few influenza cases in 1887 and/or 1888, with a notable concentration along the Baltic coast, including the capital. Significant attack rates of over ten officially registered cases per 10,000 population were reported from such widely dispersed places as the provinces of Moscow and Tver in central Russia, Irkutsk in eastern Siberia, and the city of Odessa on the Black Sea. Severe but localized epidemics were recorded in 1888 in Orenburg in the southern Urals, in 1888–1889 in portions of Tver Province, and in Moscow, Kazan, and Nizhni Novgorod in early 1889.[8] The relation, if any, between these scattered but persistent influenza flare-ups and the pandemic that developed in the last half of 1889 is unclear. The Russian events were certainly much more likely to be connected to the pandemic than the vague reports of epidemics in the spring of 1889 in the remote regions of Greenland and northern Alberta, Canada.[9] It seems probable that these two retrospective reports erroneously linked the pandemic to the respiratory ailments so common when the arrival of strangers breaks the winter isolation of far-northern outposts.

The spread of this pandemic, like the earlier ones, can be traced most easily by rising morbidity. Problems such as isolated early cases of respiratory disease later being seen as part of the pandemic and of initial phases of the pandemic escaping the attention of authorities limit the accuracy of statements on when the pandemic strain reached a particular place. A scattering of cases among travelers reaching, say, London, on a given day does not necessarily mean in any realistic sense that the epidemic began on that day. Morbidity in large groups could not be well measured anywhere except in institutions like schools, prisons, or barracks, so most writers tried to give an impression of when the number of cases began to rise dramatically in a city or region. Many estimates were, quite properly, given in terms of a given week or portion of a month. The important German writer Ripperger assigned dates to ten- or eleven-day thirds of months; Leichtenstern followed his example, and I have chosen to present onset data for Europe in the same manner in Table 4.1.

Most secondary accounts of this pandemic trace its origins to Bokhara, the capital of a Russian-dominated but still nominally independent Moslem state in what is now the Uzbek S.S.R.[10] A severe epidemic began in late May 1889 that lasted until August. Russians, Jews, and the indigenous Moslems were all affected, with total morbidity more than 50 percent. The Russian physician Heyfelder described the symptoms as high temperature for one to five days, profuse sweating, loss of appetite, malaise, nausea, vomiting, and such nervous complications as anxiety, insomnia, delirium, and depression. Overall mortality was estimated at 5,000 to 7,000 out of a population of 80,000 to 100,000, or 5.0 to 8.75 percent. The severity of the disease was blamed, on two factors: malnutrition due to a very severe winter and the month-long Ramadan fast (observed by the Moslem majority in the city); and unusually heavy concommitant Guinea worm infections caused by reduced water supplies from the previous year's drought. Heyfelder did not describe any respiratory symptoms, but later, in St. Petersburg, concluded that the cases he saw there early in the influenza epidemic were similar to those he had seen in Bokhara several months previously. He believed that the disease he saw in Bokhara was the same one that swept Russia and Europe, but did not consider that this was established beyond any doubt.[11]

There is considerable doubt about the nature of the Bokhara epidemic. Some local doctors thought that the problem was an unusually early onset of the malaria season, which certainly seems plausible. Another possibility is dengue, a mosquito-borne viral disease that was epidemic in September through October in Constantinople (Istanbul), Smyrna (Izmir), Jaffa (Haifa) and elsewhere in the eastern Mediterranean[12] and was sometimes confused with influenza during the early months of the pandemic.[13] The absence of a described rash makes dengue seem less likely, but the lack of respiratory symptoms makes influenza seem even less probable. The high death rate, summer prevalence, and the long duration of the epidemic also suggest that something other than influenza was involved. Clemow, whose writings on Russia are, as will be seen, extremely crucial, accepts Heyfelder's diagnosis, but with the important caveat that the Bokhara outbreak, like the others in Russia in 1888 and early in 1889, had no direct relationship to the true pandemic.[14] The diffusion pattern of influenza in the fall of 1889 certainly supports this view. Tessier, another contemporary foreign observer in Russia, was much more skeptical about influenza in Bokhara,[15] and Ripperger is also cautious about Heyfelder's conclusions, suggesting that both the Bokhara epidemic and the very "early" cases in St. Petersburg were really malaria.[16] In conclusion, there is little reason to believe that the origins of the 1889 virus had anything to do with events in Bokhara. If flu was there at all, malaria and other diseases must have been much more important.

It does, however, seem highly probable that, despite a retrospective claim for Chinese origins, the pandemic did in fact originate within the Russian Empire. In 1891 a report was published on influenza in Hong Kong during the months of September and October 1888. The author hypothesized subsequent spread to Russia and thence to Europe. Since half the cases had pronounced rashes,[17] the diagnosis of influenza seems doubtful, and dengue, mentioned by the author, is a real possibility. In any case, as will be described below, influenza seems to have first reached China by sea in early 1890. Although the Kirghiz people, the inhabitants of the region in Russian central Asia where the pandemic apparently did develop, sometimes called influenza "Chinese Fever," there is no evidence that they acquired the disease from China in 1889. Chinese territory was far away, the frontiers were extremely mountainous and sparsely populated, and when the pandemic did develop, it flowed from Russian territory toward, rather than away from, China.[18] A British physician, Frank Clemow, provided a detailed study of the early months of the epidemic based on careful study of unpublished official reports, including a massive study done by the Russian army. Clemow, who was in St. Petersburg when the epidemic first arrived in late October, first believed that transmission was miasmatic, as it seemed to move too quickly for person-to-person transmission.[19] He revised his views when new dates became available and after he consulted the Russian investigations, and published his conclusions in an article that, for the very first time, gave substantial evidence for a specific foyer for an influenza pandemic.[20] After noting the numerous local outbreaks around Russia in the preceding years, he located the first appearance of the pandemic in the towns of Tcheliabinsk (Chelyabinsk), in the steppe country of western Siberia, and Petropavlovsk, in what is now the northernmost portion of the Kazakh S.S.R. Both towns were struck in early October. Russian investigators suspected that Kirghiz pastoralists had the disease first and brought infection to both towns. Clemow remained unconvinced of this, noting that there was no positive evidence of prior infection

Table 4.1   The 1889–90 Pandemic in Europe

	City[a]	Onset of epidemic[b]	End of week of peak mortality (23 Nov. = 1st)[c]
Austria-Hungary	Brno (Brunn)[d]	21–31 Dec.	18 Jan. (9th)
	Budapest[e]	11–20 Dec.	11 Jan. (8th)
	Graz[f]	21–31 Dec.	
	Krakow[g]	1–10 Dec.	4 Jan. (7th)
	Linz[f]	11–20 Dec.	
	Lvov (Lemberg)[h]	21–30 Nov.	18 Jan. (9th)
	Prague	1–10 Dec.	11 Jan. (8th)
	Trieste[i]	21–31 Dec.	18 Jan. (9th)
	Vienna[f]	21–30 Nov.	28 Dec. (6th)
Belgium	Antwerp	11–20 Dec.	
	Brussels	11–20 Dec.	11 Jan. (8th)
Bulgaria	Sofia	21–31 Dec.	
Denmark	Aarhus	11–20 Dec.	
	Copenhagen	1–10 Dec.	4 Jan. (7th)
France	Bordeaux	11–20 Dec.	4, 11 Jan. (8th, 9th)
	Brest	21–31 Dec.	
	Corsica	1–10 Jan.	
	Havre	11–20 Dec.	18 Jan. (9th)
	Limoges	21–31 Dec.	18 Jan. (9th)
	Lyon	11–20 Dec.	11 Jan. (8th)
	Marseilles	11–20 Dec.	11 Jan. (8th)
	Paris	11–20 Nov.	4 Jan. (7th)
	Toulouse	21–31 Dec.	
Germany	Aachen (Aix-la-Chapelle)	21–31 Dec.	11 Jan. (8th)
	Berlin	11–20 Nov.	28 Dec. (6th)
	Bremen	21–30 Nov.	4 Jan. (7th)
	Cologne	1–10 Dec.	11 Jan. (8th)
	Gdansk (Danzig)	11–20 Nov.	28 Dec. (6th)
	Dresden	11–20 Dec.	11 Jan. (6th)
	Dusseldorf	1–10 Dec.	11 Jan. (6th)
	Frankfort-am-Main	11–20 Dec.	4 Jan. (7th)
	Hamburg	21–30 Nov.	11 Jan. (8th)
	Hanover	21–30 Nov.	28 Dec. (6th)
	Kaliningrad (Königsberg)[h]	1–10 Dec.	4 Jan. (7th)
	Kiel	1–10 Dec.	28 Dec. (6th)
	Leipzig	1–10 Dec.	11 Jan. (8th)
	Magdeburg	11–20 Dec.	11 Jan. (8th)
	Munich	1–10 Dec.	11 Jan. (8th)
	Nuremberg	11–20 Dec.	4 Jan. (7th)
	Poznan (Posen)[g]	11–20 Dec.	4 Jan. (7th)
	Strasbourg[j]	11–20 Dec.	18 Jan. (9th)
	Stuttgart	1–10 Dec.	11 Jan. (8th)
	Szczecin (Stettin)[g]	1–10 Dec.	4 Jan. (7th)
	Wroclaw (Breslau)[g]	1–10 Dec.	18 Jan. (9th)

Table 4.1 *continued*

City[a]	Unset of epidemic[b]	End of week of peak mortality (23 Nov. = 1st)[c]
Great Britain		
Belfast	1–10 Jan.	
Birmingham	21–31 Dec.	15 Feb. (13th)
Bristol	21–31 Dec.	
Cardiff	1–10 Jan.	
Channel Islands	11–20 Jan.	
Cumberland	1–10 Feb.	
Dublin[k]	21–31 Dec.	11 Jan. (8th)
Edinburgh	21–31 Dec.	18 Jan. (9th)
Glasgow	1–10 Jan.	
Hebrides	11–20 Feb.	
Leeds	1–10 Jan.	15 Feb. (13th)
Liverpool	21–31 Dec.	15 Feb. (13th)
London	11–20 Dec.	11 Jan. (8th)
Manchester	1–10 Jan.	
Nottingham	1–10 Jan.	22 Feb. (14th)
Portsmouth	11–20 Dec.	8 Feb. (12th)
Scilly Islands	11–20 Feb.	
Sheffield	1–10 Jan.	
Greece		
Athens	21–31 Dec.	
Corfu	21–31 Dec.	
Salonika	1–10 Jan.	
Iceland		
Reykjavik	July 1890	
Italy		
Bologna	21–31 Dec.	
Genoa	21–31 Dec.	
Messina	21–31 Dec.	
Milan	21–31 Dec.	
Naples	21–31 Dec.	
Palermo	1–10 Jan.	
Rome	11–20 Dec.	
Sardinia	21–31 Dec.	
Turin	21–31 Dec.	
Venice	21–31 Dec.	25 Jan (10th)
Zadar (Zara)[l]	1–10 Jan.	
Mediterranean Islands (British)		
Cyprus[m]	21–31 Dec.	
Gibraltar	1–10 Jan.	
Malta[m]	21–31 Dec.	
Montenegro[l]		
Cetinje	21–31 Dec.	
Netherlands		
Amsterdam	21–31 Dec.	18 Jan. (9th)
The Hague	21–31 Dec.	18 Jan. (9th)
Rotterdam	21–31 Dec.	18 Jan. (8th)
Norway		
"Interior"	11–20 Jan.	
Oslo (Christiana)	21–31 Dec.	25 Jan. (10th)
Portugal		
Lisbon	11–20 Dec.	11 Jan. (8th)
Porto (Oporto)	11–20 Dec.	

Table 4.1 *continued*

	City[a]	Onset of epidemic[b]	End of week of peak mortality (23 Nov. = 1st)[c]
Rumania	Bucharest	21–31 Dec.	
	Galati (Galatz)	21–31 Dec.	
Russia	Archangel	11–20 Dec.	
	Astrakhan	11–20 Nov.	
	Baku	1–10 Dec.	
	Helsinki[n]	11–20 Nov.	
	Kaluga	1–10 Nov.	
	Kazan	21–31 Oct.	
	Kharkov	11–20 Nov.	
	Kiev	11–20 Nov.	(December)
	Kuibyshev (Samara)	1–10 Nov.	
	Leningrad (St. Petersburg)	21–31 Oct.	30 Nov. (2nd)
	Moscow	21–31 Oct.	30 Nov. (2nd)
	Odessa	11–20 Nov.	14 Dec. (4th)
	Pskov	1–10 Nov.	
	Riga	1–10 Nov.	
	Rostov	21–30 Nov.	
	Saratov	1–10 Nov.	
	Sevastapol	1–10 Nov.	
	Simbirsk	1–10 Nov.	
	Tbilisi (Tifilis)	late Nov.–early Dec.	
	Turku (Abo)	11–20 Nov.	21 Dec. (5th)
	Tver	1–10 Nov.	
	Viatka	10–20 Oct.	
	Vilnius (Vilna)	21–30 Nov.	
	Warsaw[g]	11–20 Nov.	21 Dec. (5th)
Serbia[l]	Belgrade	11–20 Dec.	
Spain	Barcelona	11–20 Dec.	
	Madrid	11–20 Dec.	
	Malaga	11–20 Dec.	
	Valencia	21–31 Dec.	
Sweden	Göteborg (Gothenburg)	1–10 Dec.	4 Jan. (7th)
	Malmö	1–10 Dec.	4 Jan. (7th)
	Stockholm	21–30 Nov.	21 Dec. (5th)
	Umeå	1–10 Jan.	
Switzerland	Basel	21–31 Dec.	11 Jan. (8th)
	Bern	11–20 Dec.	4 Jan. (7th)
	Geneva	21–30 Dec.	11, 18 Jan. (8th, 9th)
	Lausanne	1–10 Jan.	11 Jan. (8th)
	Zurich	1–10 Dec.	11 Jan. (8th)
Turkey	Istanbul (Constantinople)	11–20 Dec.	

Table 4.1 *continued*

---

aModern city names are given, with older names in parentheses. Footnotes for cities/regions indicate changes in national boundaries.

bCompiled primarily from Leichtenstern, "Influenza"; Parsons, *Report*; Ripperger, *Die Influenza*; Clemow, "The Recent Pandemic"; and Linroth, *Influenza in Svedig*. For these and other references, see text notes.

cCompiled primarily from Bertillon, *La grippe à Paris*; Friedrich, *Die Influenza-Epidemie*; Linroth, *Influenza in Svedig*; Parsons, *Report*; Schmid, *Influenza in der Schweitz*; and Tessier, "L'Influenza en Russie."

dNow in Czechoslovakia.

eNow in Hungary.

f Now in Austria.

gNow in Poland.

hNow in U.S.S.R.

iNow in Italy.

jNow in France.

kNow in Ireland.

lNow in Yugoslavia.

mNow independent.

nNow in Finland.

---

among the Kirghiz, but he was interested enough to describe their way of life in some detail.

In any case, influenza spread rapidly from its initial foci. Tiumen, then the eastern railhead on the main east-west route across Siberia, was attacked on 14 October, and the disease spread eastward by foot and horseback to Irkutsk (4 December) and Chita (24 December). It moved westward along the rivers and the line of rail much more rapidly (see Map 4.1). Volga towns like Simbirsk, Samara (Kuibyshev), Saratov, and Kazan were struck in mid- to late October. Influenza advanced to the Caspian Sea at Astrakhan (in mid-November) via the Volga, and along the Ural River, to Guryev (Gurief) by early December. The disease entered the present Central Asian republics of the U.S.S.R. in two streams; eastward from the Caspian and southward from the northern steppes, reaching Tashkent, Bokhara, and Alma Ata in December and mountainous areas near the western frontier of China in January 1890. In European Russia, epidemics apparently began in St. Petersburg and Moscow at the end of October, although possible mis-diagnosis of early cases confuses the situation. The disease peaked in both cities in mid-November.[21] Kiev was hit in mid-November, as the epidemic swept from northeast to south-west across western Russia and the Ukraine.[22] As shown in Map 4.2 and Table 4.1, the Baltic region, including the Grand Duchy of Finland, was engulfed during the first three weeks of November. Baltic shipping brought the epidemic to Stockholm by

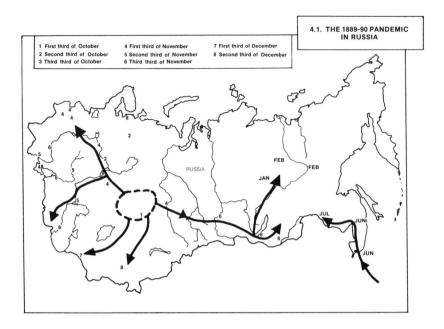

4.1. THE 1889-90 PANDEMIC IN RUSSIA

1 First third of October	4 First third of November	7 First third of December
2 Second third of October	5 Second third of November	8 Second third of December
3 Third third of October	6 Third third of November	

the end of the month.[23] Kiel, Stettin (Szczecin), Danzig (Gdansk), and perhaps Copenhagen were also attacked from the Baltic.

Infected railroad passengers brought the pandemic virus from St. Petersburg to Warsaw and Berlin, and thence to Paris and Vienna in November. In Paris, the first outbreak seems to have been among the employees of a major department store.[24] The capitals of Germany, France, and Austria-Hungary were the major foci for the subsequent diffusion of influenza along the highways, watercourses, and railroads of Europe.[25] Hannover, Hamburg, and Bremen in northwestern Germany were attacked late in November, and in December the pandemic simply exploded over almost all the Continent.

Copenhagen[26] and the ports of Malmo and Göteborg in southwestern Sweden were infected in the first days of December. The disease moved into central and southern Sweden from both Stockholm and the west coast, covering most of the country during December. A few towns in the far north escaped until January.[27] Western Germany, Switzerland,[28] Belgium, and the Netherlands[29] were all attacked during December. In France,[30] the disease radiated rapidly out of Paris, reaching Rouen,[31] Bordeaux,[32] and Marseille[33] by mid-December. Central France and Brittany lagged behind the rest of the country.[34] The first manifestation of the pandemic in Italy was probably in Rome in mid-December, no doubt as a result of rail connections. The virus reached northern Italy in two streams: along

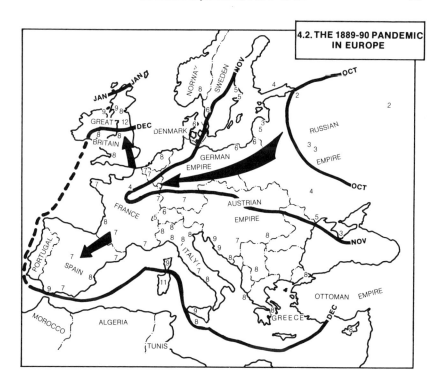

4.2. THE 1889-90 PANDEMIC IN EUROPE

1 First third of October	5 Second third of November	9 Third third of December
2 Second third of October	6 Third third of November	10 First third of January
3 Third third of October	7 First third of December	11 Second third of January
4 First third of November	8 Second third of December	12 Third third of January

the Ligurian coast to Genoa and La Spezia, and over the Austrian border toward the Adriatic.[35] Influenza had reached southern Italy, Sardinia, and eastern Sicily by the end of December. Spain and Portugal,[36] linked to Paris by rail, had flu by the middle of the month. Even in the Balkans, influenza was able to reach most major cities by rail or sea before the end of the year. Constantinople was infected about 10 December by shipping from the Black Sea ports of Russia and by trains from Vienna. The first cases were among dockworkers. The Ottoman capital was, in turn, a major diffusion center for the eastern Mediterranean, including Athens.[37] Epidemics also began in December in Cyprus and Malta.

The pandemic developed surprisingly slowly in compact, densely populated Britain. Edinburgh was infected in mid-December, supposedly by a ship from Riga, but London was the initial focus. Commuters played a major role in spreading the virus over southeastern England, and diffusion was further facilitated when Londoners dispersed to celebrate Christmas.[38] The epidemic began in mid-December in Dublin[39] and then quickly radiated out into the Irish countryside. Even though a letter from London could be delivered overnight in most towns and villages,[40] Glasgow, Belfast, and many cities in the industrial Midlands did not report epidemics until January 1890. Influenza swept over the Channel Islands in January,[41] but did not reach the Scilly Islands off the southwestern tip of England, the Hebrides off Scotland, or rural northwest England until February.

Events in Britain illustrate the importance of urban hierarchy and of accessibility for local diffusion rates. Throughout England and France, a pattern of transmission from large cities to small ones and thence to the countryside was evident to contemporary observers.[42] A similar phenomenon can be seen in the detailed reports from Sweden, the Netherlands, and Switzerland.[43] Hence, small towns and rural areas, even in compact, populous regions, often experienced influenza a month or two after the cities featured in Table 4.1 and Map 4.2. For example, in the north German province of Schleswig-Holstein, the city of Kiel was attacked very early in December, while villages only forty miles away remained free of influenza until January.[44]

Prolonged lags in outlying areas like northern Sweden, the Hebrides, western Sicily, or Iceland, which escaped until July 1890, are easy to understand, even though the epidemic did extend to such places much more rapidly than ever before. Similar lags are also evident in the Alps, where mountain villages contracted influenza weeks or even months after nearby towns in the lowlands. The Swiss villages around Zürich and Locarno are good examples.[45] Caretakers of snowbound Alpine resorts contracted influenza only after receiving visitors or going down to a town.[46] In Bergamo Province, Italy, the cities of Bergamo and Clusone had epidemics in December, while isolated villages only twenty miles away did not get influenza until February or March.[47]

The speed and volume of transatlantic shipping enabled the pandemic to become established in North America during the same month that it was sweeping over western Europe.[48] As shown in Map 4.3, Boston and New York were the earliest foci, reporting cases by mid-December. Montreal's epidemic began later in December, probably the result of an independent introduction from Europe. A report of influenza during the last ten days of December in Winnipeg, Manitoba, seems very early. The epidemic advanced rapidly westward through the American midwest, reaching St. Louis and Minneapolis by 10 January. Southward extension was also swift, with

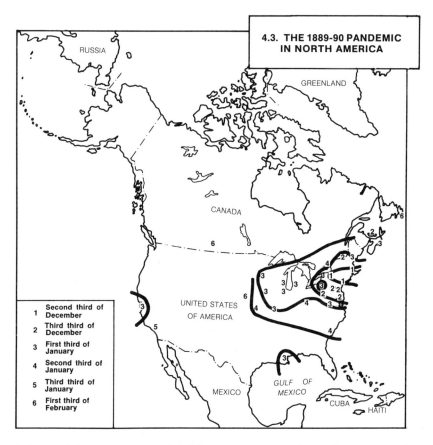

4.3. THE 1889-90 PANDEMIC IN NORTH AMERICA

1	Second third of December
2	Third third of December
3	First third of January
4	Second third of January
5	Third third of January
6	First third of February

Richmond, Virginia,[49] involved by 5 January, and Charleston, South Carolina,[50] by the middle of the month. Maritime commerce established separate foci in San Francisco,[51] New Orleans, and Halifax, Nova Scotia in early January. Unfortunately, few other details are available, but by February influenza had moved into Nebraska, Saskatchewan and, via shipping from the United States, to St. John's, Newfoundland.

Data are even sparser for Latin America, but a general pattern of a series of coastal introductions is evident on Map 4.4.[52] Mexico City may have suffered as early as mid-January; outbreaks were reported on the Gulf coast at Vera Cruz[53] and at Acapulco on the Pacific in February. Influenza was epidemic in Guatemala City by late January. On the Atlantic coast of South America, Montevideo probably was the first city struck (January);[54] Buenos Aires and Rio de Janeiro were infected in February. On the Pacific coast, ships introduced the epidemic to Chile in February,[55] to Lima and Callao, Peru, in

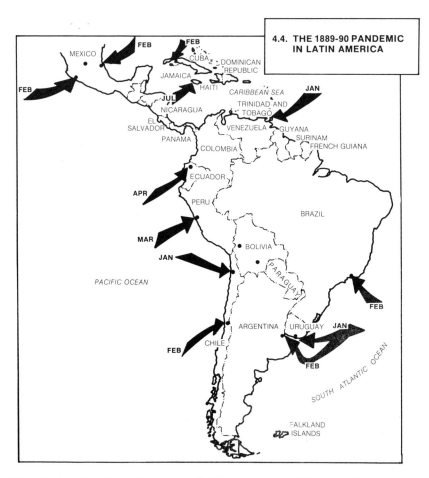

4.4. THE 1889-90 PANDEMIC IN LATIN AMERICA

March,[56] and to Ecuador in April. The progress of the pandemic was very erratic in the West Indies. Tobago and Antigua were struck in January, St. Kitts and Havana in February. Elsewhere, despite extensive inter-island shipping, there were substantial and inexplicable lags. Flu began in April in Barbados and the then-Danish Virgin Islands,[57] in June in Trinidad (four months after neighboring Tobago), and not until July in Jamaica.

A similar picture of repeated independent coastal introductions and very limited information on events in the interior is evident for Africa (Map 4.5).[58] North Africa was promptly attacked from the northern shore of the Mediterranean. In Egypt, which produced a very useful official report, epidemics began at Port Said and Alexandria in mid-December and at Cairo at the beginning of January 1890. Influenza progressed steadily down the Nile, reaching the southern frontier at Wadi Halfa by early March.[59] In January influenza began in Morocco, Tunisia, Tripoli, the Cape Verde Islands and, at the southern tip of the continent, in Cape Town.[60] From Cape Town the disease advanced by rail and road to British Basutoland (Lesotho) in late March and to Orange Free State in April. The British West African colonies of the Gambia and Sierra Leone (Freetown) were struck in mid-February; German Togo and Cameroon in late March, and various ports in the British Gold Coast (Ghana) in April[61] and May.[62] For some reason, French Senegal escaped until June. Nothing is known about influenza diffusion into the west African interior; presumably commerce along the Niger and Senegal rivers facilitated transmission.

There is even less information about east Africa. Zanzibar was struck in March, and the province of Shoa in the Ethiopian highlands did not contract the disease until November 1890. Influenza

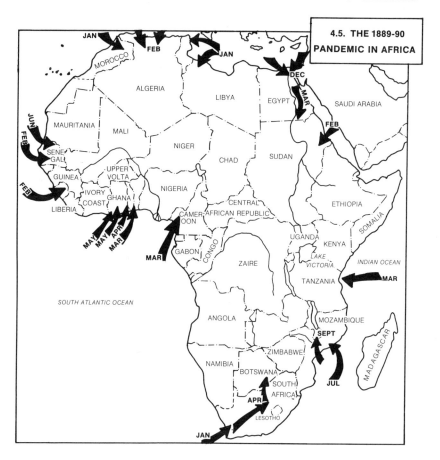

4.5. THE 1889-90 PANDEMIC IN AFRICA

was brought to the Indian Ocean islands of Mauritius and Réunion in August and September, respectively. Influenza reached the port of Quelimane in Portuguese Mozambique in July 1890 and in August advanced up the normal communications arteries, the Zambezi and Shire rivers, to reach British Nyasaland (Malawi) in September. In this extension and in subsequent local diffusion in Nyasaland, the disease followed the often-circuitous trade routes. It showed no tendency to travel cross-country and downwind on shorter routes, a strong argument against atmospheric or miasmatic transmission. Local Africans claimed, quite plausibly, that influenza had never afflicted them before and considered it a "white man's disease," one of the many consequences of European expansion.[63]

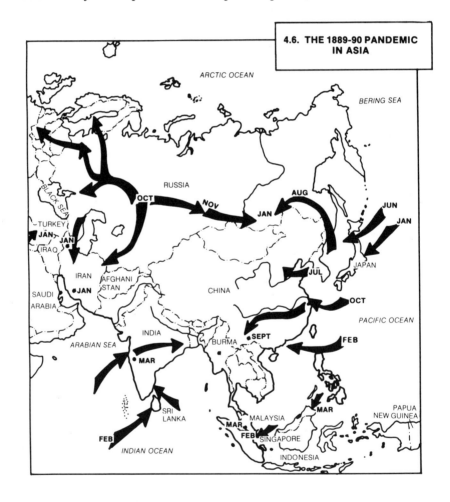

4.6. THE 1889-90 PANDEMIC IN ASIA

In Asia (Map 4.6), Persia was struck in January 1890 by influenza advancing southward from Russia on both sides of the Caspian Sea. The epidemic reached the Indian Ocean coast[64] and probably moved into what is now Pakistan, but this is the only known instance of direct overland transmission of influenza in Asia beyond the Russian Empire. Other places, including India, China, and eastern Siberia, received the virus from western Europe via oceanic trade, not from Siberia and/or Central Asia.

Beirut acquired the Mediterranean epidemic in the second half of January;[65] the Yemeni port of Hodeida was infected in early April. The virus was imported into Colombo, Ceylon (Sri Lanka), on 7 February by a British troopship from Plymouth; some rural districts on the island were still reporting cases in July. Bombay was also infected by sea in late February, with subsequent radiation over the railways to Calcutta and Madras.[66] Soldiers in Lucknow were reportedly down with flu as early as 22 February. Few other details are available for India, but influenza had reached Poona, Benares, and Meerut by mid-March and was still raging in rural Bengal in June.[67] Remote Gilgit, Kashmir, was not affected until December 1890; it was one of the last places on earth to experience the pandemic's first wave.

Singapore's epidemic began in the third week of February, and the disease was present in Malaya and British North Borneo in March. Influenza began in Japan in February. Despite Cantlie's assertion, previously discussed, that the pandemic began in Hong Kong in the fall of 1888,[68] there is no independent confirmation of influenza activity in China until 1890.[69] The disease appeared in Hong Kong in early February of that year. Local people called it "Japanese influenza,"[70] and it could have come from Japan, although direct importation from Europe seems more likely. In the north, the port of Tientsin (Tangshan) was attacked by April and nearby Peking (Beijing) by July. The remote southwestern province of Yunnan was invaded in September, apparently as a late result of influenza penetration up the Yangtze River.[71] Shanghai was reported to have had an epidemic in October,[72] a surprisingly late date for such a major port.

Australia and New Zealand were first attacked in March. Otago, a port on the South Island of New Zealand, reported cases in the first week of March. The disease was thought to have been introduced by a ship from San Francisco. Other ports, including Wellington, Dunedin, and Christchurch, were also infected in March, but Auckland, on the North Island, escaped until early May. Southeastern Australia, including Melbourne, Sydney, and the island of Tasmania, was attacked in March. Adelaide's epidemic began in mid-April,[73] and the disease began to become active in Queensland in April and at Perth, Western Australia, in May.

Eastern Siberia was, as has been described earlier, threatened by influenza advancing from the steppes of western Siberia. Moving along the route later to be followed by the Trans-Siberian Railroad, influenza spread beyond Lake Baikal to Chita by Christmas of 1889 and to Stretinsk (Sretensk) on the upper Amur River in January.[74] Here the eastward course of the disease stopped, perhaps because the Amur, used by steamers for the next segment of the route to the Pacific, was frozen. Influenza did move north to Yakutsk in February. In early June, influenza was active in Russia's Pacific bastion, Vladivostok. It appeared just after the arrival of the season's first fleet from Odessa. Sakhalin Island was also infected by steamers once the shipping season opened. Influenza then advanced westward up the Ussuri and Amur rivers to Khabarovsk in June, Blagoveshchensk in July, and finally reinfected Sretensk, the place where the winter wave had apparently died out, in August.

The fact that influenza did not traverse all of Siberia in the winter of 1889–1890, so that the far-eastern provinces of Russia were attacked from the sea, indicates the degree to which immense stretches of sparsely populated terrain can impede the spread of an acute infectious disease. Although the absence of data from Tibet, Sinkiang, Mongolia, and Manchuria makes dogmatic statements impossible, it does not appear that the highly explosive 1889–1890 virus was able to spread overland to the east with much efficiency, even on the main route across the Russian Empire. This failure suggests that earlier pandemics, like those of 1780 or 1830, would have had at least as much difficulty moving westward over the Eurasian landmass. A substantial burden of proof falls upon those who would hypothesize Chinese origins for pre-twentieth-century influenza pandemics.

The spread of the pandemic has been described thus far in terms of increased morbidity. Mortality can also be used to analyze the spatial behavior of the disease. Cause-specific mortality data are usually lacking and, when available, are problematic at best due to problems of diagnosis and multiple causes of many deaths. Total mortality by week was used by some contemporary observers, notably the French writers Tessier, Proust, and Bertillon, to chart the progress of the pandemic,[75] and dates for week of maximum mortality are given for many cities in Table 4.1. Turquan used both mortality peaks and mid-points of all flu-related deaths to chart the progress of the disease in the 87 départements of France.[76] In most cases, the maxima occurred from three to five weeks after the onset of a recognizable epidemic.

Influenza activity remained at a high level in many countries for several years after the pandemic of 1889–1890 had passed. And, as will be shown later, these episodes frequently caused higher mortality than the initial pandemic. It may be safely assumed that these outbreaks were caused by a number of distinct strains that had arisen by genetic drift from the original pandemic virus. Later epidemics have been described as "waves" of the initial pandemic, but the term is misleading if it implies a regular geographical progression. The first recurrent epidemics struck in 1890, several months after the pandemic wave, in Lisbon, Paris, Edinburgh, London, Riga, Copenhagen, Nuremberg and, in August, in Tokyo. Except for the Tokyo outbreak, none was particularly serious.[77]

Tables 4.2 and 4.3 show places affected in the second and third periods of post-pandemic outbreaks. The arrangement by months illustrates the multifocal nature of these recurrences and the fact that any diffusion was slow and local. Distribution was spotty, there was no "front" advancing from a common focus, epidemics developed more slowly and seemed to linger longer in any given place, and diffusion down the urban hierarchy was no longer the rule.[78] Winter epidemics in 1894–1895 showed similar patterns. The British observer Parsons noted that apparently "the contagium of the disease, scattered broadcast in the first epidemic, retained its vitality, but in a suspended or inconspicuous form—perhaps by transmission from one human being to another in a succession of mild sporadic cases, perhaps in some medium external to the human body—and that under the circumstances of a widely diffused character it awoke to renewed life and vigour."[79] Leichtenstern argued in similar terms, stating that influenza had simply become endemic like scarlet fever or measles, with seasonal changes in fall and spring somehow acting as a stimulus for outbreaks.[80] Prior infection gave some protection, perhaps as much as 50 percent, against attack during later waves.[81] These views, echoed by the American authority Vaughan in his important post-1918 review of influenza epidemiology,[82] seem compatible with modern ideas on pre-seeding and genetic drift.

The pandemic caused enormous morbidity in 1889 but, as in all previous and subsequent epidemics, the number of sufferers can only be guessed. Except for selected groups like soldiers in barracks or inmates of closed institutions like prisons or monasteries, whose experiences may well have been atypical, accurate attack data are not available. It was simply impossible to count all cases of a disease that was generally not severe enough to require hospitalization or a

Table 4.2   Influenza Activity, January–June 1891 ("second wave")

January	Scotland and rural areas in England
	South America (Buenos Aires, Chile)
	United States (New Orleans, Chicago, Washington, D.C., Boston, San Francisco)
	Japan (Tokyo)
February	England (Hull and scattered rural areas)
March	England (Sheffield, South Wales)
	United States (Chicago, Pittsburgh, Cleveland, Iowa, New York, Minnesota, Wisconsin, Illinois, Pennsylvania)
	Indonesia (Sumatra)
	Australia (Melbourne, Sydney)
	New Zealand (Otago)
April	London
	Christiana (Oslo)
	Göteborg
	Southern Russia
	Alsace
	Portugal
	Canada (including Vancouver Island)
	Alaska
	Washington State
May	Alaska
	Mexico City
	Copenhagen
	Russian Poland
	Cairo
June	Edinburgh
	Aberdeen

Source: Compiled from Parsons, *Further Reports* (1893), 7–8, 33–39; Leichtenstern, "Influenza," 546; Ripperger, *Die Influenza* 136, 139.

visit to a doctor. But as will be described below, a few cities did attempt to compile morbidity data. Table 4.4 shows selected morbidity estimates for a variety of places. Some figures, as for Portugal, seem impossibly high, while the percentages for Persia and Egypt can only be very rough guesses. The figures for Alexandria and Cairo show the range of estimates that local doctors could make for the same cities. One hundred and twenty-one towns and villages in Bergamo Province, Italy had estimated attack rates ranging from about a third to more than 90 percent;[83] similar variations must have been common elsewhere. While the data are sparse and impressionistic, morbidity rates in the order of one-third to one-half seem reasonable for most places.

Data on attack rates for specific age, sex, and socioeconomic groups are almost nonexistent, but most observers thought that there

Table 4.3   Influenza Activity, September 1891–February 1892 ("third wave")

September 1891	Sydney (Australia), southwestern Spain; northern Portugal; Austrian Galicia, Breslau, St. Petersburg
October	Scotland, southwest England, Kent, Londonderry (Ulster), New Zealand, Paris, Austria, Rumania, Hamburg, Lübeck, Danzig (Gdansk)
November	Belfast, Dublin, northern England, western England, southern Portugal, Budapest, Berlin
December	London, Orkney Is., Samoa, Belgium, Netherlands, Copenhagen, Stockholm, Göteborg, northern Italy, Cuba, St. Kitts, Denver, St. Louis, Philadelphia
January 1892	France, Christiana (Oslo), Bergen, New York City, Boston, Chicago, Montreal, Vancouver Is., St. John (New Brunswick), Barcelona, Santander, Granada, Greece, Sofia, Constantinople (Istanbul), Tehran, Cairo and northern Egypt, China
February	Madrid, southern Egypt
May	Argentina, Chile
July	Lima, and Tacna, Peru

Source: Compiled from Parsons, *Further Reports* (1893), 36–38; Leichtenstern, "Influenza," 547–49; Barrius, Artola, and Avenda, 125–26; M. C. Barrius, M. R. Artola, and L. Avedaño, "La epidemie de grippe habida en Lima en 1892," *La Cronica Medica* (Lima) 10(1893), pt. I, 125–26.

was little difference in vulnerability. If men and persons in certain professions were more likely to acquire the disease, it was only because they had more exposure to the public. Children and the elderly may have been, at least in some places, less susceptible than young or middle-aged adults;[84] again this may have been due to differences in exposure. Figure 4.1 shows age-specific attack rates compared to the size of age groups for Munich, where case reporting was compulsory, although doubtless incomplete. Similar curves were observed in Mainz, Hesse, and parts of Switzerland.[85] The relatively low morbidity rates among the elderly, if this was a general phenomenon, might help to explain why death rates tended to be lower during the main pandemic than in later outbreaks. The elderly were lightly hit in 1889–1890; in subsequent recurrences this vulnerable group had higher morbidity rates, resulting in higher overall mortality.

In any given community, large or small, influenza came and went fairly quickly in 1889–1890. There was a sudden rise in incidence about two weeks after the initial cases. A high level of activity was then evident for two or three weeks, followed by a rapid decline over another two or three weeks. Thus, an epidemic usually lasted from

Table 4.4   Some Morbidity Estimates, 1889-90

Place	Morbidity (percent)	Place	Morbidity (percent)
St. Petersburg[a]	50	Seine-Inférieure *Dept.*[d]	c. 40
Budapest[a]	50	Italy[e]	11
Vienna[a]	30-40	Rome[f]	50
Belgrade[a]	33	Bergamo Province[g]	33-94
Gaeta (Italy)[a]	50-77	Netherlands[h]	37.5
Portugal[a]	90	Massachusetts[i]	40
London[a]	25	Boston[j]	50
Berlin[b]	at least 33	Richmond (Virginia)[k]	40
Königsberg[b]	33	St. Louis, Mauritius[a]	67
Danzig[b]	more than 33	Peking[a]	50
Breslau[b]	30-50	Persia[l]	50
Bremen[b]	20-25	Egypt[m]	33
Cologne[b]	35-50	Alexandria[m]	33-75
Düsseldorf[b]	50-60	Cairo[m]	33-80
All Germany[b]	40-50	Constantinople[n]	33
Heligoland Island[a]	50	Santiago, Chile[o]	70
France[c]	50		

Sources:
[a]Parsons, *Report*, 109-10.
[b]Friedrich, *Die Influenza Epidemie*, 181-82.
[c]Turquan, "Statistiques," 65; based partly on extrapolation from army data.
[d]Brunon, *Grippe Dans la Seine-Inférieure*, 8; incidence higher in cities than in countryside.
[e]Giovanni Cavina, *L'influenza epidemica attraverso i secoli* (Rome, 1959), 195; reported cases only; recognized as far too low.
[f]Corradi, "L'Influenza in Italia," 392.
[g]Mora, *La Epidemia*, 14-17; range is for 121 places.
[h]Wertheim Salomonson and de Rouij, "Influenza-epidemie in Nederland," 753; based on excess deaths in general population and case/fatality rates in defined populations.
[i]George B. Shattuck, "Influenza in Massachusetts," *Boston Medical and Surgical Journal* 123 (1890); 100.
[j]A. L. Mason, "Influenza in Boston in 1889-90, Especially as it Appeared at the Boston City Hospital," *Boston Medical and Surgical Journal* 122 (1890): 147.
[k]*Virginia Medical Monthly*, 979.
[l]Tholozan, "La grippe en Perse," 251.
[m]Engel-Bey, *Influenza en Egypte*, 7, 10, 12.
[n]Limarkis, "Influenza à Constantinople," 76.
[o]Amaral, "La influenza," 96.

four to six weeks. This pattern is evident in daily case reports in Munich (Fig. 4.2), in weekly returns from three Swedish cities (Fig. 4.3), and in Swiss cantons studied by Schmid.[86]

Mortality data, systematically collected in Europe and some other places by agencies responsible for vital statistics, are much more abundant. Three indices of influenza activity are available: deaths ascribed to influenza alone, to pneumonia and/or other respiratory diseases, and, most commonly, total excess deaths.

Fig. 4.1 Age-Specific Attack Rates, Munich, 1889–1890

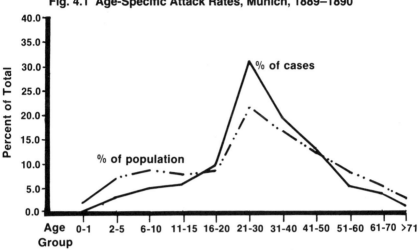

Differences in reporting criteria and the problems of assigning causes of death make overall mortality difficult to gauge, even in countries with good vital statistics. Deaths due to influenza and its complications were estimated at about 60,000 in France (1.6 per 1,000);[87] 66,000 in Germany (1.3 per 1,000)[88] and 4,500 in the Netherlands (1 per 1,000).[89] About 2,800 died in London (0.5 per 1,000),[90] 5,000 in Paris (2.5 per 1,000),[91] and 500 in Lisbon (1.6 per 1,000).[92] Some regions, like the Rhineland and portions of Austria-Hungary, were hard-hit; Belgium and Switzerland got off relatively

Fig. 4.2 Daily Case Reports in Munich, Dec. 1889–Jan 1890

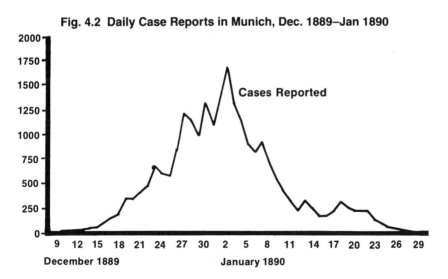

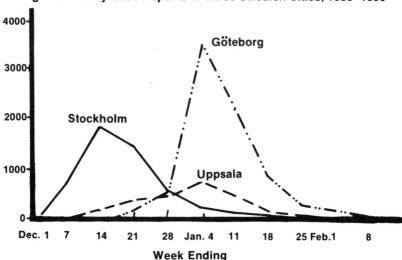

Fig. 4.3 Weekly Case Reports in Three Swedish Cities, 1889–1890

lightly. France had much higher mortality than Britain.[93] In France, rural areas had an average of 1.2 deaths per 1,000. Paris had twice that rate (2.5 per 1,000), and other urban areas 1.5 per 1,000. Disparities of 200–300 percent in nearby *départements* were very common.[94] In England and Wales rates were reported for influenza alone, so the numbers were lower; but there were also substantial regional differences. Rural Cumberland county had 0.35 influenza deaths per 1,000 people; Huntingdon reported only 0.06 per 1,000. Fifteen counties had over 0.2 flu deaths per 1,000; eleven countries had less than 0.14 per 1,000.[95] Weekly returns from other cities also show great variations, as is illustrated in Bertillon's map of northern and central Europe.[96]

While differences in reporting probably explain some of these local variations, it is clear that the lethality of influenza varied greatly from place to place in a manner that cannot be explained simply by age structure or any other factor. Regional variations make any estimate of total mortality highly speculative but, given a total population of around 360 million persons in Europe (including Russia west of the Urals), a mortality rate of 0.75 to 1 per 1,000 persons would give a figure of 270,000 to 360,000 deaths in Europe. Even a conservative suggestion that influenza killed a quarter of a million Europeans means that the toll was, as contemporary observers were fully aware, far greater than that caused by cholera or any other epidemic disease of the nineteenth century. There is no basis for estimating mortality for the rest of the world, but at least as many people must have died elsewhere. And, in the next four years, recurrences of the great pandemic took even more lives in some places than in 1889–1890.

As has been described above, the 1889–1890 virus became widely established indeed, almost endemic in many countries, resulting in localized but much more severe epidemics in the early 1890s. This was especially true in England. In London, for example, combined influenza and pneumonia death rates per 10,000 persons rose from 9.83 in 1889 to 16.5 in the pandemic year of 1890, peaked at 21.9 in 1891, and remained high at 19.8 (1892) and 20.4 (1893), before falling to 14.1 in 1894.[97] Some 5,800 persons died of influenza in London during the spring 1891 epidemic, more than twice as many as during the actual pandemic.[98] The city of Sheffield was barely struck in 1890, but hard-hit in 1891. This case, admittedly extreme, is shown in Figure 4.4. Figures for Chicago (Fig. 4.5) give a similar picture; later epidemics, especially that of 1891, caused far more excess deaths than occurred in 1890. In Massachusetts, it was the third wave, in late 1891 to early 1892, whose mortality exceeded that of the original pandemic (Fig. 4.6). Ireland had more than twice the 1890 flu death rate two years later, in 1892 (Fig. 4.14).[99] In Switzerland, however, the mortality of 1889–1890 exceeded all other years, being rivaled only by a severe outbreak in 1893–1894 (Fig. 4.7).

Fig. 4.4 Weekly Flu Mortality in Sheffield, England, 1890–1893

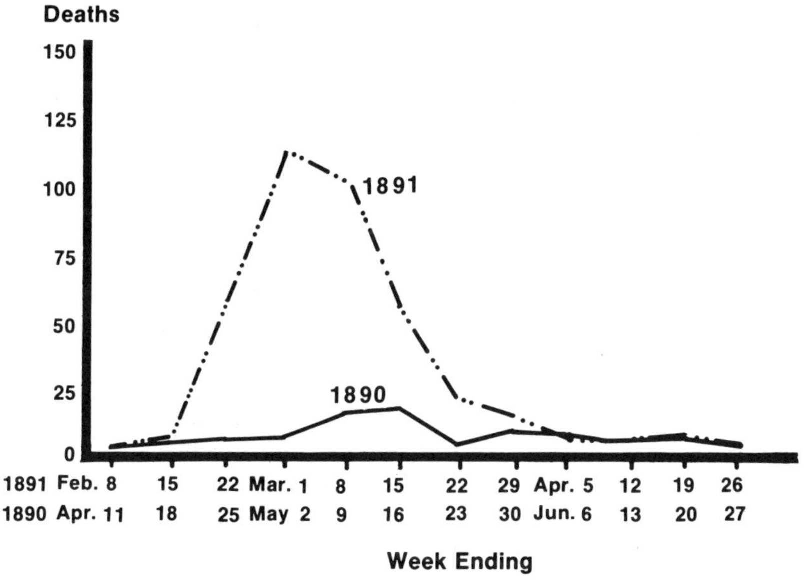

Week Ending

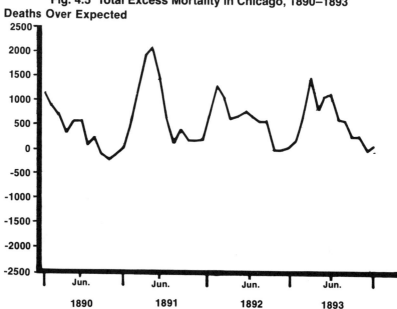

Fig. 4.5 Total Excess Mortality in Chicago, 1890–1893

Mortality in this pandemic and in its recurrences was, like every other pandemic discussed in this work, closely linked with secondary pneumonia and/or other respiratory diseases and was worst among the elderly. Virtually every study cited in this chapter, from Kiev[100] to Nyasaland,[101] mentions much higher age-specific mortality among the elderly. Careful documentation of this is provided in Denmark[102] and in the Dutch, German, and Swedish studies cited above; even the Egyptian data show a similar pattern although, as might be expected in a poor tropical country, the tremendous number of infant and toddler deaths gives a strong peak for younger years that probably has little direct connection with influenza.[103]

A few examples will illustrate age-specific death rates in 1889–1890 and subsequent years. Figure 4.8 is from Bertillon's detailed study of the 1889–1890 epidemic in Paris. Mortality rose with age for both sexes; the higher rate for younger males could represent higher attack rates for men and/or greater incidence of concomitant diseases. In England and Wales, men were also more susceptible than women at ages under sixty-five.[104] Swiss returns, however, frequently show higher female mortality at lower ages as well as among the elderly for the entire period 1889–1890 to 1894. Age-specific rates for both sexes for deaths ascribed to influenza alone in England and Wales show a heavy bias toward the elderly, both in

Fig. 4.6 Flu and P–I Death Rates in Massachusetts, 1887–1904

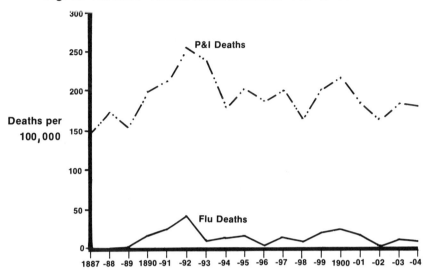

1890 and the more lethal year of 1891 (Fig. 4.9). Finally, Figures 4.10 and 4.11 show a similar pattern for pneumonia-influenza deaths in London for 1889, which may be taken as a base year, and for four subsequent years of intense influenza activity. The markedly higher

Fig. 4.7 Influenza-Related Deaths in Switzerland, Nov. 1889–Oct. 1894

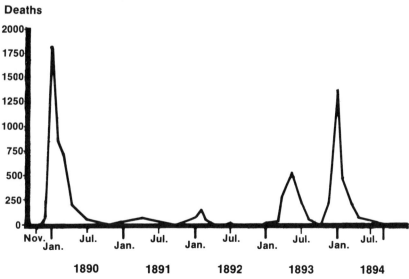

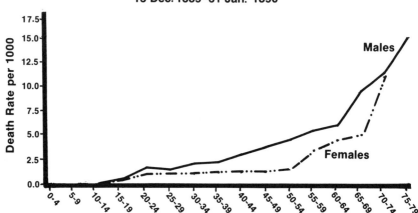

**Fig. 4.8 Influenza Deaths by Age and Sex in Paris,
15 Dec. 1889–31 Jan. 1890**

rates among older people after 1890 may, as noted earlier, have
resulted from greater morbidity among the elderly in the second and
later recurrences of influenza.

The age distribution of influenza-related deaths in 1889–1890 and
later waves is quite typical of every pandemic save that of the fall of
1918. As in 1957 and 1968, the initial wave of the 1889 pandemic
was often less lethal than later ones. Indeed, if the virus of the mild
spring wave of 1918 was in fact closely related to the deadly fall

**Fig. 4.9 Influenza Death Rates by Age, England and Wales,
1890 and 1891**

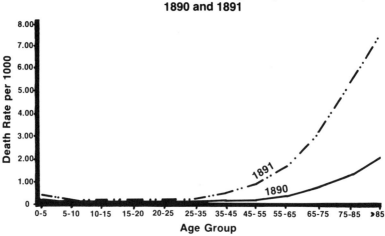

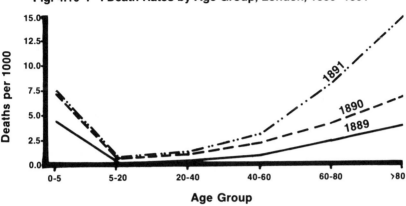

Fig. 4.10 P–I Death Rates by Age Group, London, 1889–1891

strain, this mild initial-wave–severe second-wave pattern may be a common feature of modern pandemics. Unless the episode of 1837 is seen as a late wave of the 1833 pandemic, this was a new phenomenon in 1889, suggesting that the advent of modern transportation systems facilitated recurrent waves of modified viruses of the pandemic strain.

There was another flurry of influenza activity during the winters of 1899–1900 and 1900–1901. The pandemic status of these outbreaks is, as will be discussed below and in chapter 5, germane to theories of antigenic recycling suggested by serological studies. This outbreak, whatever its nature, was not a dramatic event like the pandemics previously described and has not usually been seen as a

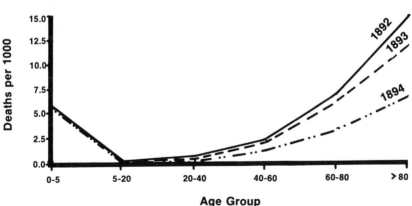

Fig. 4.11 P–I Death Rates by Age Group, London, 1892–1894

pandemic.[105] It showed no obvious geographical spread, was clinically mild, and attracted little notice in the medical literature. Indeed, were it not for a survey conducted by the United States Public Health Service and increases in pneumonia-influenza death rates recorded in several countries, the epidemic would probably have gone almost unnoticed.

Some centers of flu activity for the two winters in question are shown in Table 4.5. The data are clearly incomplete. For example, influenza must have been active in the western United States in 1899–1900. The Alaskan outbreak of June 1900 came from the "lower 48" and, in conjunction with a measles epidemic that spread from northeastern Siberia, caused heavy mortality among Aleut and other indigenous populations.[106] Norfolk Island, hundreds of miles off the Pacific coast of Australia, was attacked in September 1900 as a result of shipping from Australia,[107] so influenza must have been present there during the Southern Hemisphere winter. Case reports from Göteborg also suggest that influenza was prevalent in Sweden in 1899 as well as 1900 (Fig. 4.12). The geographical patterns of influenza diffusion in these years are not at all clear.

If the Cuban report is dismissed as incorrect or not linked to the main outbreak, the data are consistent with a picture of influenza prevalence in parts of northwestern Europe in late 1899, with spread in Europe and to the United States and perhaps to Australia in the early months of 1900. London and Belfast were struck in December, with flu becoming widespread in England, Ireland, and Scotland during the first weeks of 1900.[108] The disease was also widespread in Amsterdam around the beginning of the year, and Denmark was attacked in late 1899 and early 1900.[109] Rome and northern Italy were heavily attacked by the end of January,[110] and France was

Fig. 4.12 P–I Deaths Among the Elderly, England and Wales, 1897–1902

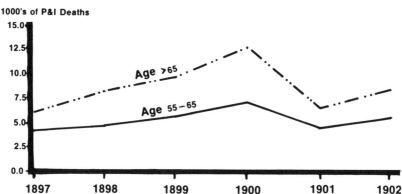

1000's of P&I Deaths

Table 4.5   Influenza Activity, 1899–1901

Date	Place	Date	Place
December 1899	Matanzas, Cuba	December 1900	Copenhagen
	London		Alexandria
	Belfast		Mexico City
	La Rochelle, France		San Luis Potosi, Mexico
January 1900	Edinburgh		Albuquerque, N.M.
	Cork, Dublin		Detroit
	Dover		Madrid
	Liverpool	January 1901	New Haven, Conn.
	Northern Italy		Boston
	Rome		Albany, N.Y.
	Netherlands		Richmond, Va.
March 1900	Malta		Denver
	Lima		Davenport, Iowa
	Massachusetts		Dubuque, Iowa
	France		Indiana
June	Western Alaska		New Orleans
September	Norfolk Island		Grand Rapids, Mich.
	(off Australia)		Biloxi, Miss.
October	Milwaukee		Binghamton, N.Y.
	Los Angeles		Buffalo, N.Y.
November 1900	Millburn, N.J.		Providence, R.I.
	Cincinnati		Corpus Christi, Tex.
	Memphis		Wilmington, Del.
	El Paso, Tex.		Beaufort, N.C.
	Juarez, Mexico		Prague
	Toledo, Ohio		Puerto Rico
December 1900	Chicago		Dublin
	Portsmouth, N.H.		Trieste
	Philadelphia		Astoria, Ore.
	Champaign, Ill.		Belgium
	Bangor, Maine		Honolulu
	New York		Louisville, Ky.
	New Bern, N.C.		Juneau, Alaska
	Columbus	by March 1901	Turkey
	Pittsburgh	June–July	Australia
	Sioux Falls, S.D.		
	Peoria, Ill.		
	Baltimore		
	Omaha		
	Utah		
	Nogales, Ariz.		
	British Columbia		
	Japan		
	Kingston, Ontario		
	Toronto		

Source: Compiled from sources given in notes 106–13.

experiencing widespread but mild flu by early March.[111] The advance of the epidemic in Europe was suspended during the summer, but epidemics occurred in the winter of 1900–1901 in places like Prague, Trieste, and Madrid, which had hitherto escaped. The Madrid outbreak, which began in December 1900, caused very high morbidity but, as elsewhere, mortality rates were low.[112] Massachusetts had an epidemic in March 1900, and pre-seeding must have occurred elsewhere in North America during the summer. The data in Table 4.5, largely drawn from information compiled by the U.S. Public Health Service, indicate sudden fall to early winter flare-ups in scattered foci in the United States, Canada, and Mexico. In Australia, the epidemic of mid-1901 caused especially high morbidity among children.[113]

As noted above, case returns from Göteborg indicate widespread influenza activity there in late 1899 (Fig. 4.13). Influenza death returns for the city of London show, in addition to the serious recurrences of the 1889–1890 pandemic, a sharp rise in deaths in 1899 before the peak year of 1900 (Fig. 4.6). The flu of 1899–1901 was, as usual, most lethal among the elderly. Combined pneumonia-influenza deaths for two older age groups are shown in Figure 4.14 for England and Wales; again it is clear that the epidemic was active in 1899 and was almost as lethal as in 1900. Data from Massachusetts, one of the relatively few American states with good mortality reporting, show noticeable peaks for both pneumonia and influenza deaths in early 1899 as well as in March 1900. In Ireland, however, there was no peak in 1899, but a dramatic jump in influenza-specific mortality in 1900 (Fig. 4.15).

Fig. 4.13 Influenza Cases in Göteborg, Sweden, 1889–1900

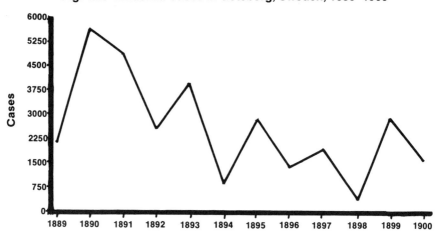

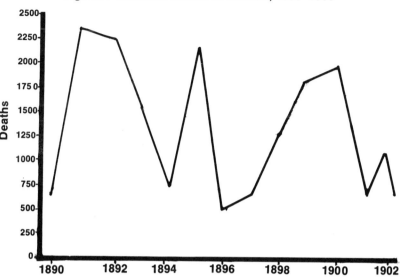

Fig. 4.14 Influenza Deaths in London, 1890–1903

The data, however patchy, do suggest a notable surge in influenza and influenza-related deaths in the period 1899–1901, with a "first wave" in late 1899 to early 1900 in Europe and North America. The returns from Massachusetts suggest, however, extensive prevalence of influenza in the early months of 1899, so the origins remain hypothetical. Elevated mortality suggests a possible pandemic, but clear geographical patterns are not evident. Perhaps this is because of deficient information and/or extensive pre-seeding. The epidem-

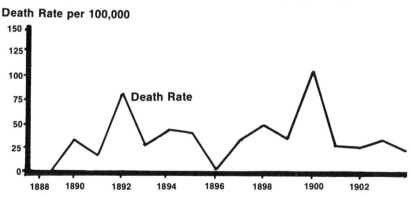

Fig. 4.15 Influenza Death Rates in Ireland, 1888–1904

82   *Pandemic Influenza*

ics of 1899–1901 could represent a last gasp of the 1889–1890 pandemic.

Sero-archeological studies have suggested that strains similar to the H2N2 virus of 1957 circulated in the late nineteenth century, and that this was followed by a virus similar to the H3N2 pandemic strain of 1968.[114] A circa 1890 date is plausible for the H2N2 strain; and if the theory is correct, there must have been an H3N2 between then and 1918. The best possibility is that an H3N2 virus, a novel type, was active at the turn of the century and caused, by definition, a true pandemic, but a pandemic that probably was not discernible from morbidity and mortality reports alone. The mild nature of the 1899–1901 flu could have been due to residual immunities among the older people who had survived 1889–1890; probably only the H antigen was new.

5
Overview and Conclusions

Pandemics of influenza are infrequent events; since 1700 there have been only three to five a century. Table 5.1 lists pandemics and possible pandemics from the eighteenth century to the present. It is evident that pandemics, and hence antigenic shifts in the influenza A virus, occur at irregular intervals. There is no chronological pattern that would allow us to predict when a new outbreak might come, and pandemics show no correlation with war, peace, depressions, or periods of economic boom. Twice, in the 1730s and in the 1830s, one pandemic followed almost on the heels of another. On the other hand, the pandemics of 1781, 1830, and 1889 developed about half a century after the previous ones. Intervening years were not, of course, free from influenza; genetic drifts of prevailing strains resulted in substantial local activity and fairly sizable epidemics in many nonpandemic years.

The geographical origins of influenza pandemics have been the subject of speculation for centuries. As for so many epidemic diseases, there was a xenogenic assumption—it came from *somewhere else*. Western writers of the eighteenth and nineteenth centuries tended to look eastward, to Russia and beyond, for the origins of major influenza epidemics.[1] This was an old tradition; Europeans

Table 5.1 Pandemics and Probable Pandemics Since 1700

	Years since last pandemic	Place of origin or of first report	Viral type
1729–30	?	Russia (?)	(?)
1732–33	2	Russia	(?)
1781–82	48	Russia; China (?)	(?)
1788–89(?)	6	Russia	(?)
1830–31	41–48	Russia; China	(?)
1833	2	Russia	(?)
1836–37(?)	3	Russia (?)	(?)
1889–90	52–56	Russia	H2
1899–1900	9	(?)	H3
1918	18	France, USA	H1N1(Hsw1N1)
1957	39	China	H2N2
1968	11	China	H3N2
1977	9	China	H1N1

had long feared the arrival of disasters such as the Mongols, Turks, and the plague from shadowy regions in the east. The march of cholera from India via Iran and Russia in the 1820s and 1830s did not surprise them. Russia, a vast and backward empire, was frequently cited as the breeding ground for influenza. Epidemics seemed to spread westward from Russia, and Europeans felt justified in referring to influenza as "Russian flu."[2] 1889-90

A second tendency, existing in the nineteenth century and probably strengthened by Clemow's work on the 1889 pandemic, described in chapter 4, has been to look eastward of European Russia. Who really knew, even in St. Petersburg or Moscow, what went on in the immense lands beyond the Volga? As Norris has written in a discussion of the geographical origins of plague, Europeans had long held fears "in the context of which almost any unfavorable manifestation could be attributed to the region of Central Asia."[3] In 1928, Gill asserted that "all authorities are agreed that pandemics of influenza can almost invariably be traced to 'the silent spaces' of Asia, Siberia, and China."[4] His views have been echoed by later writers, including Andrewes[5] and Beveridge.[6]

Recent opinion on the birthplaces of pandemics has, however, shifted from the sparsely populated expanses of Central Asia to China. The virulent fall wave of the 1918 pandemic probably originated in France or, possibly, the United States, but the other twentieth-century pandemic strains, those of 1957, 1968, and 1977, have all emerged in China.[7] Indeed, as described in chapter 1, studies on domestic ducks and other farm animals suggest that southern China is a likely place for interspecies virus recombination. The intensive production of ducks in this densely populated region seems to provide excellent conditions for the appearance of pandemic strains. Such recombinants are the most likely source of new strains, and southern China may be the influenza epicenter for recent decades.[8] By extrapolation, Chinese origins could easily be postulated for earlier pandemics. Indeed, early outbreaks in China were reported for both the 1781 and 1830 pandemics.

Nevertheless a general theory of an epicenter in China encounters two problems, one recent and one historical. The 1977 virus first appeared in northern China and subsequently spread over the world. But as pointed out in chapter 1, it was identical to an H1N1 strain that had circulated in 1950. There are three possible explanations of how the virus could have avoided normal genetic drift.[9] It could have existed in a dormant state in man, although there is no evidence that this is possible. Alternatively, it could have existed unchanged in an animal host. A human lung parasite, presumably the fluke *Paragonimus westermani*, has been hypothesized for this role, but again there is no evidence to support such a mechanism. The third possibility is that the 1950 viruses were literally frozen, in a laboratory or in nature. A human icebox seems more plausible than a glacier or the Arctic ice cap. Although it is reported that there was no work being done in China on H1N1, there has been considerable speculation that the 1977 virus escaped from a laboratory.[10] At any rate, the mysterious origins of the 1977 pandemic and the fact that it was first discovered in northern China reduce the number of pandemics that can be traced to Shortridge and Stuart-Harries' postulated south China epicenter to two, 1957 and 1968. Their very attractive hypothesis fits well with current views on the natural history of the virus, but not with the historical evidence.

The other argument against Chinese origins for pre-twentieth-century pandemics has been discussed in connection with the 1889 pandemic. It is difficult to see how influenza could have reached Russia and western Europe from China. A sea route, even in stages, seems most implausible and could hardly explain how Russia was the proximate source for spread westward. Overland transport seems marginally more likely, but still presents grave difficulties. Norris's argument in regard to the spread of plague in the fourteenth century is applicable to influenza as well. "Theories of rapid, extensive, and covert movement of the disease through the human population in sparsely-inhabited areas along the trade routes of Asia" must be viewed with great caution.[11] Even in 1889–1890, flu advanced over Siberia very slowly, and China was attacked by sea from western Europe, not overland from Central Asia. While it is impossible to exclude Chinese origins for the pre-1889 pandemics, transmission to Europe seems so difficult that it is hard to imagine it happening once, let alone for every pandemic. Of the pandemics described here, the 1830 outbreak is the most likely to have followed this route.

Where did these pre-twentieth-century pandemics originate, if not in China? Of course, there may well be more than one place of origin; it seems unlikely that they all developed in the same region. India cannot be excluded; its dense population might have harbored an assortment of viral strains and, as the cholera outbreak of the 1820s demonstrated, a disease could move overland from India to Russia, and thence sweep across western Europe and reach the Western Hemisphere. The Americas seem very unlikely candidates, at least prior to 1918, and Africa is excluded. But perhaps the European identification of Russia was correct after all. Influenza was usually first reported in Moscow, St. Petersburg, or some other city in European Russia; perhaps pandemic strains at least sometimes developed in the Russian heartland. Or, if the events of 1889 can be generalized, there could be, or could have been, a nursery of novel strains of influenza A virus in the broad region of what is now southwestern Siberia, northern Kazakhstan, and the steppe country of Russia between the Volga and the Urals. This region, a bit more precisely defined than Gill's "silent spaces" or Beveridge's suggested "hinterland of the Eurasian landmass,"[12] would fit the historical data better than south China, even if conditions in China seem, on the basis of our present knowledge of the ecology of the virus, more favorable for the creation of pandemic strains.

Detailed research in local archives in China and the U.S.S.R. could shed light on the origins and early diffusion of pandemics, as could new knowledge of the distribution and behavior of the virus. Meanwhile, the problems of where and how pandemics develop must remain open.

Influenza generally spread from east to west across Europe. Southern Scandinavia and the Baltic region were usually attacked early, Spain and Italy late and from the north and northeast, with the Pyrenees and the Alps acting as partial barriers. Cities clearly were foci of diffusion in several pandemics, and dissemination down the urban hierarchy was probably a general phenomenon. Two exceptions to the rule of east-west movement are discussed in chapter 3. In 1837 there was a strong north to south movement, but an east-west component can be detected as well, and in any case this may not have been a true pandemic. The nonpandemic 1847 outbreak, like the apparent pandemic of 1580 and the epidemic of 1709, spread from the Mediterranean northward into Europe. North America consistently seems to have been attacked from Europe via North Atlantic shipping, although sometimes, as in 1732 and 1789, with one-year lag.

At no time did the rate of spread exceed the speed of human travel, which for most of the period was by foot, horse, or sail. Influenza was, of course, spread much more rapidly in 1889 than ever before, through railroad and steamship travel. The pandemics of 1781 and 1830 moved at a more leisurely pace than the others. In all of these pandemics, diffusion patterns fall into the "massive frontal" model proposed by Pyle and Patterson.[13]

Epidemics of influenza are most common in cold weather. Pandemics, including those since 1957 and most of those discussed here, have followed this trend. This is not an invariable rule however, as the mild wave of 1918 spread in the spring, and the deadly second wave began in late summer. The outbreaks of 1729, 1832,

1833, 1837, and 1889 took place in fall and winter. There was extensive spring and summer activity in 1782, 1789, and 1831. But there were major lulls in the summers of 1831 and 1833, before the pandemic resumed its advance in southern Europe.

Pre-seeding, the quiet establishment and maintenance of a new virus with a low, perhaps unnoticed level of activity in a population, has long been discussed by epidemiologists. Disseminated viruses can then burst forth in a sudden epidemic when conditions become favorable. Thus, the onset of cold weather might trigger a sudden epidemic in a large area with no obvious diffusion pattern.[14] As was shown in Houston in the 1970s, activity of a new viral type at the end of one influenza season can be a "herald wave," anticipating off-season pre-seeding and emergence of that type in epidemic form during the next winter.[15] The diffusion of the 1957 and 1968 pandemics can be explained in these terms. Epidemic in the Southern Hemisphere winter, they reached North America and Europe during the same months. Early isolations heralded the pandemic strain, which diffused quietly during the Northern Hemisphere summer and, thus pre-seeded, burst out in the Northern Hemisphere with the opening of schools and the onset of cold weather.[16] There is no proof that earlier pandemics spread in this fashion, but pre-seeding must have been widespread in 1900; and the events of 1836–1837, described in chapter 3, could be interpreted as the sudden winter emergence of a new virus that had become widely established in Europe during the warmer months. Similarly, quiet spread of a pandemic strain could have occurred in eastern Europe during the summer of 1729 and in southern Europe during the summer lulls in the advances of the 1831 and 1833 pandemics.

In view of the current interest in the roles of birds and mammals such as pigs, horses, turkeys, and wild and domestic ducks in the ecology of the influenza A virus,[17] it is interesting to note that ideas of close connections between animal and human influenza are quite old. Concurrent epidemics among humans and animals, usually horses, are frequently mentioned in the early literature.[18] Horses were, of course, kept in large numbers in the pre-automobile era and lived in close contact with people in both rural and urban areas.

Horses were said to have been attacked before people in England during the 1732–1733 pandemic.[19] During a 1775 outbreak in London, Fothergill wrote that "horses and dogs were much affected; those especially that were well kept. The horses had severe coughs, were hot, forbare eating, and were long in recovering. Not many of them died that I heard of; but several dogs." Hounds suffered more severely than other breeds.[20] In the same year, horses and dogs in

Exeter and in Dorset also seemed to contract influenza, sometimes before people did.[21] Exeter horses again had "colds" during the pandemic of 1782, but dogs and cattle remained healthy.[22] Benjamin Rush saw apparent flu cases in two cats, two dogs, and one horse in Pennsylvania during the 1789–1790 outbreak.[23] Animal cases of what seemed to be influenza were widely reported in England in 1803. Cows, dogs, and horses were common victims; cats suffered in Shrewsbury and very fatal local epizootics attacked pigs as well.[24] Horses at Penang, Malaya, "were very subject to colds" during the 1831 pandemic.[25] Widespread equine "flu" was noted by a London veterinarian in 1833.[26] "Catarrhal and rheumatic affections" were described in Prussian cattle and horses during the 1837 epidemic,[27] and these animals were also thought to have contracted influenza in two districts in France in the same year.[28] In 1889–1890, when apparent equine influenza was again seen in England, there was considerable speculation on possible relations with the human disease. Most doctors and veterinarians were skeptical. Horses and other animals seemed vulnerable to a number of different flulike ailments, none of which was necessarily the same as the human disease, and epizootics often did not coincide with epidemics.[29]

The historical record can shed little light on the role of animals in the epidemiology of influenza. Lack of information on a possible connection to ducks is not surprising, since ducks harbor the virus in their gastrointestinal tracks without showing obvious symptoms. It is certainly possible that some early reports of epizootics, especially among horses, refer to genuine sharing of a virus by man and animals; but in that case, any impact on the spread or severity of pandemics is doubtful. Of course, domestic animal reservoirs could have been sources of viruses in interpandemic years. Although Kilbourne has suggested that the barnyard may be the graveyard rather than the nursery of human strains,[30] we cannot rule out the possibility that animals like horses might play a role in the appearance of new pandemic strains. Could this have happened in the steppes of southeastern Russia or Kazakhstan?

The paucity and unreliability of statistics, as described in earlier chapters, make it impossible to speak with any precision about morbidity or mortality rates during past pandemics, but it is known that all were characterized by high morbidity and low case-mortality rates. Contemporary observations suggest that something in the order of 25 to 50 percent of any given population contracted influenza during a pandemic. Age, sex, and socioeconomic status made little or no difference in incidence rates; everyone was vulnerable to attack.

Influenza mortality rates, whether expressed as case-mortality or total death rates, were always low. If data for 1889 are indicative, overall rates of up to 1 percent and case-mortality rates ranging from 0.5 percent to more than 2 percent were normal. In all the pandemics described here, deaths were mostly among the elderly. None of them caused anything like the level of mortality experienced in 1918, and none produced the high death rates among young adults that characterized that disaster.

It is possible that useful mortality figures, especially age-specific data, could be gleaned from the parish registers kept in countries like England or Sweden for centuries prior to the advent of civil registration. Since influenza passes quickly through any given population, monthly tallies would be more valuable than annual death totals. Hope-Simpson has attempted to use early parish registers for Gloucestershire, England, to study influenza epidemics.[31] The English registers, however, do not give cause of death, and his assumptions that specific mortality peaks were caused by influenza are suspect. The massive Cambridge University study of English population history shows very little correlation between high-mortality "crisis" years and influenza epidemics. Even when influenza was present, famine and other diseases may have caused most of the excess deaths.[32]

The toll from earlier pandemics was, however, very substantial. Thousands—or more likely hundreds of thousands—died whenever a new strain swept Europe and, as nineteenth-century writers were well aware, influenza epidemics regularly killed many more people than died during the dreaded incursions of cholera. Cholera caused great suffering, killed a high percentage of its victims, and struck people of all ages. Outbreaks of the disease caused panic, social upheaval, medical controversies, and brought about public health reforms; it mesmerized contemporaries and has, understandably, attracted much attention from medical historians.[33] Cholera, however, attacked only a small proportion of any given population. Influenza, on the other hand, struck millions of people, causing widespread illness and temporary disruption, but individual sufferers had little reason to fear death. It quietly killed old people by the thousands, but caused much less alarm and had a much smaller impact on society than cholera or many other contagious diseases.

Viral antigenic types for 1889 and subsequent pandemics are shown in Table 5.1. Direct observations have been possible since 1957, but determinations for episodes preceding the isolation of the virus in 1933 have depended upon a technique known as sero-archaeology. Antibodies against virus surface antigens, especially hemagglutinin, persist for decades in the blood. Thus, immunological studies of stored sera and of elderly persons can show what types of virus have infected them in the past. Specimens collected before 1957 from persons born before 1889 frequently have antibodies against the H2 antigen. People born at the end of the century do not have this antibody, so H2 viruses must have disappeared by then. Similarly, persons tested before the 1968 pandemic who were born in the late 1890s often retain antibodies against H3; people born twenty years later lack this, so an H3 virus must have circulated from about 1899 to circa 1918. Recent studies have suggested that an H1N1 strain became active about a decade before 1918.[34] Unfortunately, barring the unlikely discovery of usable sera collected in the nineteenth century, this method can give no information on pandemics prior to 1889.

Sero-archaeological investigations conducted in the Netherlands, Japan, the United States, and other countries have led to a theory of antigenic recycling.[35] That is, only a few potential pandemic serotypes exist, and they reappear at intervals of many decades, when population immunity levels have declined. The dramatic reemergence of H1N1 in 1977 has cast some doubt on the existence of such long-term cycles,[36] but the whole 1977 episode is so unusual, perhaps even artificial, that it may have little bearing on the antigenic recycling theory.

Periods of prevalence of influenza A subtypes since 1889 are shown in Table 5.2. Pandemics introduced new subtypes, which underwent years of antigenic drift until they were replaced by new ones. H3N2 has continued to co-circulate with H1N1 since 1977. Recent evidence suggests that the same situation prevailed in 1908–1917, prior to the deadly "swine flu" virus of 1918. This had led to a revival of earlier predictions by Masurel and co-workers that an

Table 5.2   Periods of Prevalance of Virus Subtypes

Subtype	Period
H2	1889-1898
H3	1899-1917
H1N1	1908-1957
H2N2	1957-1968
H3N2	1968-Present
H1N1	1977-Present

Source: Noble, "Epidemiological and Clinical Aspects," in Beare, ed., Influenza Research, 20; Masurel and Heijtink, "Recycling of H1N1," 397-401.

Unfortunately, the historical record can do little to support or contradict the fascinating theory of periodic reappearance of a limited number of antigenic types. Diffusion patterns and morbidity-mortality data do not provide evidence on the subtypes responsible for eighteenth- and early nineteenth-century pandemics and, in the absence of virological information, no identification can be made. It is obvious that the old H2 antigens must come from 1889, since there was no other pandemic for a half-century before it. H3 must be associated with the events of 1899–1900; indeed, sero-archaeological evidence for a new subtype confirms that this obscure episode was in fact a true pandemic.

Several conclusions emerge from this study. Pandemics, whether defined by geographical/clinical criteria or by virology, occur at irregular intervals, which give little credence to notions of periodicity or predictability. Notions of eleven- or sixty-eight-year cycles are untenable.[38] Geographical origins of pandemics seem most likely to be in eastern Russia–central Asia and, at least since 1957, in China; further research might shed more light on this problem. Pandemics have always spread in patterns consistent with the speed and pathways of human travel. Since 1889, they have been able to move much more quickly and have reached virtually every inhabited place on earth. Rapid long-distance travel makes possible the inter-hemispheric pre-seeding observed during the middle months of 1957 and 1968. Certainly, the historical record gives no support to views that the virus is widely dispersed in a dormant state in a population, ready to burst forth with changes in solar radiation or other environmental stimuli.[39] It is also unnecessary to hypothesize viral visitors from outer space.[40] High morbidity and low mortality, with most deaths among the elderly, were characteristic of all eighteenth- and nineteenth-century epidemics. The absence of virological data for early years limits what can be learned about possible antigenic recycling, but the timing of the pandemics of the late nineteenth century is consistent with recent theories.

Perhaps the single most striking generalization confirmed by this study is similarity among most pandemics, and the utter uniqueness of the 1918 outbreak. No other pandemic spread so explosively, killed nearly as many victims, nor caused remotely as much mortality among young and middle-aged people. Predicting a new pandemic is like predicting an earthquake in California or Japan; the exact time is doubtful, but a prognosticator can be sure that one will come within a few decades. The 1918 pandemic was, so far, a singular event, and any recurrence is impossible to forecast.

Notes

Chapter 1

1. "Changes in Premature Mortality—United States 1982–1983," *Morbidity and Mortality Weekly Report* 34, no. 2 (Jan. 18, 1985): 17–18.

2. Edwin O. Jordan, *Epidemic Influenza: A Survey* (Chicago, 1927), 214, citing Bureau of Census estimates.

3. *Ibid.*, 214–18.

4. K. David Patterson, "The Demographic Impact of the 1918–19 Influenza Pandemic in Sub-Saharan Africa: A Preliminary Assessment," in *African Historical Demography*, vol. 2., ed. C. Fyfe and D. McMaster, (Edinburgh, 1981), 401–31.

5. F. M. Burnet, "Portraits of Viruses: Influenza Virus A," *Intervirology* 11 (1979): 203.

6. High virulence might have been caused by the particular virus and/ or concomitant bacteria. See Kingsley M. Stevens, "The Pathophysiology of Influenzal Pneumonia in 1918," *Perspectives in Biology and Medicine* 25 (1981): 115–25, for a recent hypothesis.

7. World Health Organization, "A Revision of the System of Nomenclature for Influenza Viruses: A WHO Memorandum," *Bulletin of the World Health Organization* 58 (1980): 585–91.

8. G. R. Noble, "Epidemiological and Clinical Aspects of Influenza," in *Basic and Applied Influenza Research* ed. A. S. Beare, (Boca Raton, Fl., 1982), 12; W. I. B. Beveridge, *Influenza: The Last Great Plague: An Unfinished Story of Discovery* (New York, 1977), 17; E. D. Kilbourne, "Influenza Pandemics in Perspective," *Journal of the American Medical Association* 237 (March 21, 1977): 1225–27.

9. R. G. Webster and W. G. Laver, "The Origin of Pandemic Influenza," *Bulletin of the World Health Organization* (hereafter *Bulletin WHO*) 47 (1972), 449–52; D. J. Alexander, "Ecological Aspects of Influenza A Viruses in Animals and Their Relationship to Human Influenza: A Review," *Journal of the Royal Society of Medicine* 75 (1982): 799–811; V. S. Hinshaw and R. G. Webster, "The Natural History of Influenza A Viruses," in *Basic and Applied Influenza Research*, ed. Beare, 79–104.

10. G. G. Schild, "Influenza," in *A World Geography of Human Diseases*, ed. G. M. Howe (London, 1977), 343; P. Palese and J. F. Young, "Variation of Influenza A, B, and C Viruses," *Science* 215 (March 19, 1982); 1470; A. P. Kendall, G. R. Noble, J. J. Skehel and W. R. Dowdle, "Antigenic Similarity of Influenza A (H1N1) Viruses from Epidemics of 1977–1978 to 'Scandinavian' Strains Isolated in Epidemics of 1950–1951," *Virology* 274 (1978): 632–36.

11. Noble, "Epidemiological and Clinical Aspects of Influenza," 18–20;

N. Masurel, "Serological Characteristics of a 'New' Serotype of Influenza A Virus: The Hong Kong Strain," *Bulletin WHO* 41 (1969): 461–68; N. Masurel and W. M. Marine, "Recycling of Asian and Hong Kong Influenza Virus Hemagglutinins in Man," *American Journal of Epidemiology* 97 (1973): 40–49.

12. K. D. Patterson and G. F. Pyle, "The Diffusion of Influenza in Sub-Saharan Africa During the 1918–1919 Pandemic," *Social Science and Medicine* 17 (1983): 1299–1307.

13. Alfred W. Crosby, Jr., *The Columbian Exchange: Biological and Cultural Consequences of 1492* (Westport, Conn., 1972).

14. Kilbourne, "Influenza Pandemics in Perspective," 1227.

15. K. F. Shortridge and C. H. Stuart-Harries, "An Influenza Epicentre?" *Lancet* 2 (October 9, 1982): 812–13; K. F. Shortridge, "Pandemic Influenza: Application of Epidemiology and Ecology in the Region of Southern China to Prospective Studies," in *The Origin of Pandemic Influenza Viruses,* ed. W. G. Laver, (New York, 1983), 191–97.

16. A. Villard, *Leçons cliniques à propos de l'épidémie de 1889 et 1890* (Paris, 1890), 106; W. T. Vaughan, *Influenza: An Epidemiologic Survey* (Baltimore, 1921), 60–61; C. A. Gill, *The Genesis of Epidemics and the Natural History of Disease* (New York, 1928), 223; G. F. Pyle and K. D. Patterson, "Influenza Diffusion in European History: Patterns and Paradigms," *Ecology of Disease* 2 (1984): 173–84.

17. See, for example, Vaughan, *Influenza;* F. M. Burnet and E. Clarke, *Influenza: A Survey of the Last Fifty Years in the Light of Modern Work on the Virus of Epidemic Influenza* (Melbourne, 1942); Beveridge, *Influenza: The Last Great Plague;* E. D. Kilbourne, "Epidemiology of Influenza," in *The Influenza Virus and Influenza,* ed. Kilbourne (New York, 1975), 483–538.

18. See, for example, Richard Collier, *The Plague of the Spanish Lady: The Influenza Pandemic of 1918–19* (New York, 1974); and A. W. Crosby, Jr., *Epidemic and Peace, 1918,* (Westport, Conn., 1976). There is still plenty of work to be done on 1918.

19. Richard Fiennes, *Zoonoses of Primates: The Epidemiology and Ecology of Simian Diseases in Relation to Man* (Ithaca, N.Y., 1967), 130.

20. Burnett, "Portrait of a Virus," 210; and general discussion in Frank Fenner, "The Effects of Changing Social Organization on the Infectious Diseases of Man," in *The Impact of Civilization on the Biology of Man,* ed. S. V. Boyden, (Toronto, 1970), 48–68.

21. William H. McNeill, *Plagues and Peoples* (Garden City, N.Y., 1976), 69–97.

22. Kwang-Chih Chang, *The Archaeology of Early China,* 3d ed., (New Haven, Conn., 1977), 167; Wang Zhongsheu, *Han Civilization* (New Haven, 1982), 57; Robert J. Wenke, *Patterns in Prehistory: Mankind's First Three Million Years* (New York, 1980), 271. I am grateful to Dr. Janet E. Levy for advice on this subject.

23. August Hirsch, *Handbook of Geographical and Historical Pathology,* vol. 1, (London, 1883), 7.

24. A. Ripperger, *Die Influenza: Ihre Geschichte, Epidemiologie, Aetiologie, Symptomatologie und Therapie* (Munich, 1892), 18.

25. Pyle and Patterson, "Influenza Diffusion in European History," 176–77.

26. Hirsh, *Handbuuk*, vol. 1, 7–9; Ripperger, *Die Influenza*, 18–47; Gottleib Gluge, *Die Influenza oder Grippe* (Minden, 1837), table opposite p. 43.

27. O. Leichtenstern, "Influenza," in *Malaria, Influenza, and Dengue*, ed. J. Mannaberg and O. Leichtenstern (Philadelphia, 1905), 525–26; G. Olagüe de Ros, "La epidemia europea de gripe de 1708–1709," *Dynamis* 1 (1981): 53–55; R. Sisley, *Epidemic Influenza: Notes on Its Origin and Method of Spread* (London, 1891), 3; J. C. Saillant, *Tableau historique et raisonné des épidémies catarrhales* (Paris, 1780), 63.

28. Saul Jarcho, "Yellow Fever, Cartography, and the Beginning of Medical Geography," *Journal of the History of Medicine and Allied Sciences* 25 (1970): 131–42; Gary P. Shannon, "Disease Mapping and Early Theories of Yellow Fever," *Professional Geographer* 33 (1981): 221–27.

29. W. P. Glezen, "Serious Morbidity and Mortality Associated with Influenza Epidemics," *Epidemiological Reviews* 4 (1982): 25–44.

30. See, for example, Noble, "Epidemiological and Clinical Aspects of Influenza," 33–36; Schild, "Influenza," 360.

31. Gluge, *Die Influenza*.

Chapter 2

1. For introduction to 18th-century medical and epidemiological thought, see, among others, Lester S. King, *The Medical World of the Eighteenth Century* (Chicago, 1958); C-E. A. Winslow, *The Conquest of Epidemic Disease: A Chapter in the History of Ideas* (Princeton, 1944); and Richard H. Shryock, "Germ Theories in Medicine Prior to 1870: Further Comments on Continuity in Science," *Clio Medica* 7 (1972): 81–109. For relevant discussion of early 19th-century epidemiological theories, see Erwin H. Ackerknecht, "Anticontagionism Between 1821 and 1867," *Bulletin of the History of Medicine* 26 (1948): 562–93; recent arguments in John M. Eyler, *Victorian Social Medicine: The Ideas and Methods of William Farr* (Baltimore, 1979), 97–99; and Margaret Pelling, *Cholera, Fever and English Medicine, 1825–1865* (Oxford, 1978), 16–18, 298–303. John Farley shows that the best scientific evidence of the 1820s favored the spontaneous generation of parasitic worms in "The Spontaneous Generation Controversy (1700–1860): The Origin of Parasitic Worms," *Journal of the History of Biology* 5 (1972): 95–125. His point is directly relevant to early disputes among "miasmatists" and "contagionists"; it is dangerous to evaluate past science by deciding what was more nearly correct in terms of modern knowledge.

2. For general discussion, see Erwin H. Ackerknecht, *Therapeutics from the Primitives to the Twentieth Century* (New York, 1973), esp. 78–91; and Guenther B. Risse, "Epidemics and Medicine: The Influence of Disease on Medical Thought and Practice," *Bulletin of the History of Medicine*, 53 (1979), 505–19.

3. Most of the contemporary articles cited in this chapter discuss therapy, often at great length.

4. Representative lists of pandemics are given in August Hirsch, *Handbook of Geographical and Historical Pathology*, vol. 1 (London, 1883), 18; A. Ripperger, *Die Influenza: Ihre Geschichte, Epidemiologie, Aetiologie, Symptomatologie und Therapie* (Munich, 1892), 140; Warren T. Vaughan, *Influenza: An Epidemiologic Study* (Baltimore, 1921), 6–11; and W. I. B. Beveridge, *Influenza: The Last Great Plague: An Unfinished Story of Discovery* (New York, 1977), 27–30.

5. Sources for this epidemic are Olagüe de Ros, Guillermo, "La epidemia europea de gripe de 1708–9," *Dynamis* 1 (1981): 51–86; Hirsch, *Handbook*, 9; and Ripperger, *Die Influenza*, 47–48.

6. Sources are Hirsch, *Handbook*, 9; Ripperger, *Die Influenza*, 49–50; Gottleib Gluge, *Die Influenza oder Grippe* (Minden, 1837), 71–73; and Ditmar Finkler, "Influenza," in *Twentieth Century Practice: An International Encyclopedia of Modern Medical Science*, vol. 15 (New York, 1898), 21–22.

7. Unless otherwise cited, data are from Gluge, *Die Influenza*, 73–78; Hirsch, *Handbook*, 9; Ripperger, *Die Influenza*, 50–53; and Alfonso Corradi, "Annali delle epidemie occorse in Italia dalle prime memorie fino al 1850," *Memorie della Società medico-chrurgica di Bologna*, vol. 6, fasc. 6 (1876), 1374.

8. Charles-Jacques Saillant, *Tableau historique et raisonné des épidémies catarrhales vulgairement dites la grippe depuis 1510 jusques et y compris celle de 1780* (Paris, 1780), 25.

9. Charles Creighton, *A History of Epidemics in Britain*, 2d ed., vol. 2. (London, 1985), 343.

10. Thomas B. Peacock, *On the Influenza or Epidemic Catarrhal Fever of 1847–8* (London, 1848), 108.

11. *Gazette médicale de Paris*, "Recherches sur la grippe de l'Europe et celle de Paris," 2d sér., vol. 1 (1833), 329; Finkler, "Influenza," 22.

12. Giovanni Cavina, *L'influenza epidemica attraverso i secoli* (Rome, 1959), 106–8; Edward F. G. Martiny, *Die Influenza oder Grippe: eine contagios-epidemische Krankheit* (Weimar, 1835), 9.

13. John Hjaltelin, "On the Epidemic Influenzas of Iceland, Especially the Last One of 1862," *Edinburgh Medical Journal* 8 (Feb. 1863): 697.

14. Noah Webster, *A Brief History of Epidemic and Pestilential Diseases*, vol. 1 (Hartford, Conn., 1799), 230; John Duffy, *Epidemics in Colonial America* (Baton Rouge, 1953), 191.

15. Duffy, *Epidemics in Colonial America*, 192–93.

16. Hirsch, *Handbook*, 9.

17. *Gazette médicale de Paris*, "Recherches," 329.

18. As argued by Gluge, *Die Influenza oder Grippe*, 78; Ripperger, *Die Influenza*, 50; Finkler, "Influenza," 22.

19. Heidenreich, "Om Influenza," *Tidskrift för Läkare och Pharmaceuter* 2 (1833), 177; and Georg F. Most, *Influenza Europaea oder die Grösseste Krankheits-Epidemie der neueren Zeit* (Hamburg, 1820), 44.

20. Gluge, *Die Influenza oder Grippe*, 78.

21. Ibid., 77.

22. J. A. F. Ozanam, *Histoire médicale générale et particulière des maladies épidémiques, contagieuses et épizootiques qui ont régné en Europe depuis les temps les plus reculés jusqu' à nos jours,* 2d ed., vol. 1 (Lyon, 1835), 134.

23. Saillant, *Tableau historique,* 26.

24. E. A. Wrigley and R. Schofield, *The Population History of England, 1541–1871* (Cambridge, Mass., 1981), 338–39.

25. Ripperger, *Die Influenza,* 51–52.

26. Ozanam, *Histoire médicale,* 1st ed., vol. 1 (1817), 313.

27. This supersedes an earlier interpretation of the 1729 and 1732 pandemics by Gerald F. Pyle and K. David Patterson, "Influenza Diffusion in European History: Patterns and Paradigms," *Ecology of Disease* 2 (1984): 177.

28. Major sources are Hirsch, *Handbook,* 9; Ripperger, *Die Influenza,* 53–55; Heinrich Schweich, *Die Influenza: ein Historischer und Atiologischer Versuch* (Berlin, 1836), 81–85; and John Arbuthnot, "An Essay Concerning the Effects of Air on the Human Body" (London, 1751), in *Annals of Influenza or Epidemic Catarrhal Fever in Great Britain from 1510 to 1837,* ed. Theophilus Thompson, (London, 1852), 36–37.

29. Ozanam, *Histoire médicale,* vol. 1, 138; Ripperger, *Die Influenza,* 53.

30. B. Maugue, "Dissertation sur les rhumes épidémiques qui ont régné pendant l'hiver 1732 et continué dans le mois de janvier 1733," *Revue d'Hygiène et Thérapie* 8 (1896): 118 (publication of a 1733 manuscript).

31. "Medical Observations in Edinburgh," reprinted in Thompson, *Annals,* 40.

32. John Huxham, *Observations on the Air and Epidemical Diseases* (London, 1758); translated from Latin and reprinted in Thompson, *Annals,* 33.

33. Cavina, *L'influenza epidemica,* 108.

34. Webster, *A Brief History,* vol. 2, 35.

35. J. Fuster, *Monographie clinique de l'affection catarrhale* (Montpellier, 1861), 383.

36. Gluge, *Die Influenza oder Grippe,* 81.

37. Ripperger, *Die Influenza,* 53.

38. Personal Communication from Dr. Ann Jannetta, 26 June 1985, based on Japanese chronicles. I am grateful to Dr. Jannetta, who is working on the history of epidemics in Japan, for this and other references to influenza in that country.

39. "Medical Observations," in Thompson, *Annals,* 41; Huxham, "Observations," in Thompson, *Annals,* 32; Mauge, "Dissertation sur les rhumes," 118; Ripperger, *Die Influenza,* 54; Finkler, "Influenza," 22.

40. Ozanam, *Histoire médicale,* 1st ed., vol. 1 (1817), 138; Huxham, "Observations," in Thompson, *Annals,* 35; "Medical Observations," in Thompson, *Annals,* 41.

41. Ozanam, *Histoire médicale,* 2d ed., vol. 1 (1835), 145–46.

42. Creighton, *History of Epidemics,* vol. 2, 346.

43. "Medical Observations," in Thompson, *Annals,* 41.

44. Hirsch, *Handbook*, 9.

45. Ibid.; Finkler, "Influenza," 24–25; Ripperger, *Die Influenza*, 57; Corradi, "Annali delle epidemie," 1401.

46. Hirsch, *Handbook*, 10; Ripperger, *Die Influenza*, 58–59.

47. Vaughan, *Influenza*, 12; M. Webster Brown, "Early Epidemics of Influenza in America," *Medical Journal and Record* 135 (4 May 1932): 449. Beveridge, *Influenza*, 28, considers it a possible pandemic. Basic sources are Finkler, "Influenza," 26–27; Hirsch, *Handbook*, 10; Ripperger, *Die Influenza*, 60–61; Ozanam, *Histoire médicale*, 2d ed., vol. 1 (1835), 165–69.

48. George Baker, *De Catarrho et de Dysenteria Londinensi Epidemicus utrique an. 1762* (London, 1769), trans. in Thompson, *Annals*, 75.

49. Ozanam, *Histoire médicale*, 2d ed., vol. 1 (1835), 165.

50. Baker, *De Catarrho*, in Thompson, *Annals*, 75, n. 1.

51. Ibid., 75, in reference to diffusion in England.

52. Hirsch, *Handbook*, 10; Ripperger, *Die Influenza*, 61–62.

53. Hirsch, *Handbook*, 10; Ripperger, *Die Influenza*, 62–64; Anthony Fothergill, "An Account of Epidemic Catarrh (Termed Influenza), as it Appeared at Northampton, and in the Adjacent Villages, in 1775," *Memoirs of the Medical Society of London* 3 (1792), 30; Richard Pearson, *Observations on the Epidemic Catarrhal Fever, or Influenza, of 1803; To Which Are Subjoined Historical Abstracts Concerning the Fevers of 1762, 1775, and 1782*, 2d ed. (London, 1803), 16.

54. Saillant, *Tableau historique*, 93, noting the presence of influenza in Paris in January 1780.

55. Hirsch, *Handbook*, 10–11; "An Account of the Epidemic Disease Called the Influenza of the Year 1782, Collected from the Observations of Several Physicians in London and in the Country, by a Committee of the Fellows of the Royal College of Physicians in London," *Medical Transactions*, vol. 3 (1785), 61.

56. Webster, *A Brief History*, vol. 1, 268; vol. 2, 33.

57. "An Account of the Epidemic," 61.

58. Edward Grey, "An Account of the Epidemic Catarrh of the Year 1782; Compiled at the Request of a Society for Promoting Medical Knowledge," *Medical Communications* 1 (1784); 4. This study and the one reported in "An Account of the Epidemic" depended heavily on responses to questionnaires sent out to physicians.

59. Basic sources are Schweich, *Die Influenza*, 114–16; Gluge, *Die Influenza oder Grippe*, 93–107; Hirsch, *Handbook*, 11; Ripperger, *Die Influenza*, 65–71.

60. Gray, "An Account of the Epidemic Catarrh," 4.

61. "An Account of the Epidemic," 55, says 20 May, but another contemporary observer states that flu reached Edinburgh around 1 June. See William Scott, "An Account of the Influenza as It Appeared in Northumberland in the Months of June and July 1782," *Medical Communications* 5 (1783–85), 261. Either date is possible; the later one would fit a little better with reports from Glasgow (1st week of June) and Musselburgh, a small town a few miles east of Edinburgh (9–10 June). For these dates, see "An Account of the Epidemic," 56.

62. E.g., Hirsch, *Handbook*, 11; Ripperger, *Die Influenza*, 69; Finkler,

"Influenza," 30–31; Pyle and Patterson, "Influenza Diffusion in European History," 178–79.

63. "An Account of the Epidemic," 55.

64. John Clark, "A Letter to Dr. Leslie, F.R.S., on the Influenza; As It Appeared at Newcastle-upon-Tyne," in P. Dugud Leslie, *An Account of the Epidemical Catarrhal Fever, Commonly Called Influenza, as It Appeared in the City and Environs of Durham, in the Month of June, 1782* (London, 1783), 83–84.

65. Scott, "Influenza . . . in Northumberland," 257.

66. Details on the diffusion of the epidemic in Britain are given in "An Account of the Epidemic," 55–56; Scott, "Influenza . . . in Northumberland," 257, 261; Clark, "A Letter to Dr. Leslie," 83–84; Leslie, *Influenza . . . in Durham*,31–33; R. Hamilton, "Some Remarks on the Influenza That Appeared in the Spring of 1782," *Memoirs of the Medical Society of London* 2 (1794), 429–30; B. Parr, "An Account of the Influenza as It Appeared in Devonshire in May 1782," *Medical Commentaries* 5 (1783–5), 251; William Falconer, *An Account of the Epidemic Catarrhal Fever, Commonly Called the Influenza, as It Appeared at Bath, in the Months of May and June, 1782* (Bath, 1782), 8–12; John Haygarth, "Of the Manner in Which the Influenza of 1775 and 1782 Spread by Contagion in Chester and Its Neighbourhood," in Thompson, *Annals*, 193; D. Monro, "Account of the Late Influenza," *Medical Commentaries* 5 (1783–85), 248; Arthur Broughton, *Observations on the Influenza or Epidemic Catarrh; as It Appeared in Bristol and Its Environs During the Months of May and June, 1782* (London, 1782), 5.

67. Haygarth, "Of the Manner," 193; Leslie, *Influenza . . . in Durham*, 53.

68. Ozanam, *Histoire médicale*, 2d ed., vol. 1 (1835), 184.

69. Cavina, *L'influenza epidemica*, 145.

70. Schweich, *Die Influenza*, 116.

71.. Gray, "An Account of the Epidemic Catarrh," 4; Peter Irving, *An Inaugural Dissertation on the Influenza* (New York, 1794), 10–11.

72. M. Pétrequin, "Recherches pour servir à l'histoire générale de la grippe de 1837 en France et en Italie," *Gazette médicale de Paris*, 2d sér., vol. 5 (1837), 802. His translation was "catarrh chinois."

73. Schweich, *Die Influenza*, 114–15.

74. H. Haeser, *Geschichte der Medizin und der epidemischen Krankheiten* (Jena, 1882), 948.

75. Martiny, *Die Influenza oder Grippe*, 14.

76. Dr. Ann Jannetta, personal communication.

77. Webster, *A Brief History*, vol. 1, 268–69; vol. 2, 33–35.

78. Fuster, *Monographie clinique*, 408.

79. Gluge, *Die Influenza oder Grippe*, 103.

80. "An Account of the Epidemic," 57.

81. Parr, "Influenza . . . in Devonshire," 251.

82. Scott, "Influenza . . . in Northumberland," 261.

83. Broughton, "Influenza . . . in Bristol," 6.

84. E.g., Falconer, *Influenza . . . at Bath*, 8; "An Account of the Epidemic," 56–57, 70; Leslie, *Influenza . . . in Durham*, 40; Ozanam, *Histoire médicale*, 2d ed., vol. 1 (1835), 185.

85. Gray, "An Account of the Epidemic Catarrh," 4.

100   Notes

86. Fothergill, "Epidemic Catarrh . . . at Northampton," 39.

87. Sir Macfarlane Burnet and David O. White, *Natural History of Infectious Disease*, 4th ed. (Cambridge, 1972), 205–6.

88. Beveridge, *Influenza*, 13.

89. Vaughan, *Influenza*, 12; Ripperger, *Die Influenza*, 140.

90. Basic sources are Schweich, *Die Influenza*, 122; Gluge, *Die Influenza oder Grippe*, 108–11; Hirsch, *Handbook*, 11; Ripperger, *Die Influenza*, 73–74.

91. Samuel F. Simmons, "Of the Epidemic Catarrh of the Year 1788," *London Medical Journal* 9 (1788): 337–38, quoting an issue of the *Gazette Salutaire* (Paris) not available to me.

92. Klaus Linroth, C. Wallis, and F. W. Warfvinge, *Influenza in Svedig* (Stockholm, 1890), v.

93. Simmons, "Epidemic Catarrh . . . of 1788," 335.

94. Vaughan May, "Observations on the Influenza, as It Appeared at Plymouth in the Summer and Autumn of the Year 1788," *Medical Commentaries*, 2d. decade, vol. 7 (1794), 478–79.

95. George Bew, "Of the Epidemic Catarrh of the Year 1788," *London Medical Journal* 9 (1788): 354–55.

96. Simmons, "Epidemic Catarrh . . . of 1788," 343–44.

97. "Maladies qui ont régné à Paris pendant le mois d'août 1788," *Journal de médecine, chirurgie et pharmacie* 77 (Paris, 1788): 102.

98. Boucher, "Maladies qui one régné à Lille dans le mois de septembre 1788," *Journal de médecine, chirurgie et pharmacie* 77 (1788): 288; Taranget, "Constitutions épidémiques observées à Douay en Flandre," *Journal de médecine, chirurgie et pharmacie* 77 (1788): 451.

99. Gluge, *Die Influenza oder Grippe*, 111.

100. John Warren, "Letter to Dr. Lettsom," 30 May 1790, in Thompson, *Annals*, 199.

101. William Currie, "A Short Account of the Influenza Which Prevailed in America in the Year 1789," *Transactions of the College of Physicians of Philadelphia*, vol. 1 (1793), 150–51.

102. Taylor and Hansford, untitled note, in William Currie, *A Historical Account of the Climates and Diseases of the United States of America* (Philadelphia, 1792), 332.

103. Webster, *A Brief History*, vol. 1, 289.

104. Warren, "Letter to Dr. Lettsom," 199.

105. Webster, *A Brief History*, vol. 1, 289.

106. Benjamin Rush, "An Account of the Influenza as It Appeared in Philadelphia in the Autumn of 1789, in the Spring of 1790, and in the Winter of 1791," in his *Medical Inquiries and Observations*, 3d ed., vol. 2 (Philadelphia, 1809), 444.

107. John Lindsay, "An Account of the Epidemic Catarrh of the Latter End of the Year 1789, as It Appeared in Jamaica," *Medical Commentaries*, 2d. decade, vol. 7 (1793), 506.

108. C. Chisholm, "Observations on the Influenza, as It Appeared in the West Indies," *Medical Commentaries*, 2d. decade, vol. 5 (1790), 326–28.

109. Rush, "Influenza . . . in Philadelphia," 447–48. I can find no further information on Spanish America.

110. Webster, *A Brief History*, vol. 1, 291; Irving, *An Inaugural Dissertation*, 11.

111. Ripperger, *Die Influenza*, 73.

112. Simmons, "Epidemic Catarrh . . . of 1788," 337.

113. Ibid., 339.

114. Bew, "Catarrh of the Year 1788," 364.

115. "Maladies . . . à Paris," 102.

116. Taylor and Hansford in Currie, *A Historical Account*,322.

117. Currie, "A Short Account," 151.

118. Chisholm, "Influenza . . . in the West Indies," 326–28.

119. Lindsay, "Epidemic Catarrh . . . in Jamaica," 526.

120. Simmons, "Epidemic Catarrh . . . of 1788," 352.

121. Currie, *A Historical Account*, 405–6.

122. Gluge, *Die Influenza oder Grippe*, chart opposite 42; Hirsch, *Handbook*, 7–9.

Chapter 3

1. Summaries are given in the surveys by Erwin H. Ackerknecht, *A Short History of Medicine* (Baltimore, 1982), 145–56; and Richard H. Shryock, *The Development of Modern Medicine* (Madison, 1974), 109–247.

2. Ralph Cuming, one of the doctors surveyed by Beddoes (see n. 9 below) estimated that 9 out of 10 British physicians were anti-contagionists. He may overstate the case, but a strong majority of Beddoes's 124 respondents were opposed to the theory of contagious spread of influenza.

3. Richard Dunning, "Mr. Dunning on Influenza," *Medical and Physical Journal* 10 (1803): 139–40.

4. Representative discussions are given in Henry H. Porter, *An Account of the Origin, Symptoms, and Cure of the Influenza or Epidemic Catarrh* (Philadelphia, 1832), 9–12; Jules Guerin, "Observations sur l'épidémie de Paris," *Gazette médicale de Paris* 2 (1831): 217–19; J. A. Hingeston, "On the Late Influenza," *London Medical Gazette* 17 (1833): 199–201; and J. A. F. Ozanam, *Histoire médicale générale et particulière des maladies épidémiques, contagieuses et épizootiques qui ont régné en Europe depuis les temps plus reculés jusqu' à nos jours*, 2d. ed., vol. 1 (Lyon, 1835), 25–31. A British observer noted that, in contrast to most of his fellow M.D.s, the British public considered influenza contagious. William Brown, "Notice of the Late Influenza in Edinburgh," *Edinburgh Medical and Surgical Journal* 43 (1835): 31–32.

5. See, for example, A. C. Baldwin, "An Account of the Influenza of 1831–2 as It Appeared in Burke County, Georgia," *American Journal of Medical Sciences* 11 (1832–33): 34–36; H.-C. Lombard, "Quelques observations sur la grippe qui a régné à Genève en 1831," *Gazette médicale de Paris*, 2d sér., vol. 1 (1833): 730–32; and George Fyfe, *Observations on Influenza, Its Nature and Consequences, as It Appeared in the Author's Practice, During Its Recent Prevalence in Newcastle-upon-Tyne, and at Former Periods in Edinburgh* (Newcastle-upon-Tyne, 1833), 13–21. Many of the articles cited in this chapter include extensive discussions of therapy.

6. George Rosen, *A History of Public Health* (New York, 1958), 192–293; James H. Cassedy, *American Medicine and Statistical Thinking, 1800–1860* (Cambridge, Mass., 1984); and John M. Eyler, *Victorian Social Medicine: The Ideas and Methods of William Farr* (Baltimore, 1979).

7. Basic sources are August Hirsch, *Handbook of Geographical and Historical Pathology*, vol. 1 (London, 1883), 12; A. Ripperger, *Die Influenza: Ihre Geschichte, Epidemiologie, Aetiologie, Symptomatologie und Therapie* (Munich, 1892), 74–75; Georg Friedrich Most, *Influenza Europea oder die Grösseste Krankheits-Epidemie der neuren Zeit* (Hamburg, 1820), 75–77; and Heinrich Schweich, *Die Influenza: ein historischer und ätiologischer Versuch* (Berlin, 1836), 127–28.

8. Gerald F. Pyle and K. David Patterson, "Influenza Diffusion in European History: Patterns and Paradigms," *Ecology of Disease* 2 (1984): 179–80; Ripperger, *Die Influenza*, 77–78; Hirsch, *Handbook*, vol. 1, 12; Theophilus Thompson, *Annals of Influenza or Epidemic Catarrhal Fever in Great Britain from 1510 to 1837* (London, 1852), 202–4; Richard Pearson, *Observations on the Epidemic Catarrhal Fever, or Influenza, of 1803* 2d. ed., (London, 1803), 33–46.

9. Thomas Beddoes collected 124 reports from British practitioners and published summaries in *Medical and Physical Journal* no 10 (1803): passim.

10. Gherardino Michele, *La grippe ossia descrizione della malattia catarrale attualmente dominante* (Milan, 1803), 3.

11. John Herdman, *A Plain Discourse on the Causes, Symptoms, Nature and Cure of the Prevailing Epidemical Disease Termed Influenza* (Edinburgh, 1803), 4.

12. W. I. B. Beveridge, *Influenza: The Last Great Plague: An Unfinished Story of Discovery* (New York, 1977), 29.

13. Data from Hirsch, *Handbook*, vol. 1, 13; Ripperger, *Die Influenza*, 79.

14. Shadrach Ricketson, *A Brief History of the Influenza Which Prevailed in New York in 1807* (New York, 1808), 3–4.

15. Gottlieb Gluge, *Die Influenza oder Grippe* (Minden, 1837), 136. For an earlier and less detailed treatment of this and other outbreaks, see Patterson, "Pandemic and Epidemic Influenza, 1830–1848," *Social Science and Medicine* 21, no. 5 (1985): 571–80.

16. Gluge, *Die Influenza*, 136; George Bennett, "On the Epidemic Catarrh, or Influenza, Which Prevailed at Manila," *London Medical Gazette* 8 (1831): 523–25.

17. Bennett, "Influenza . . . at Manila," 525.

18. Ibid., 523.

19. Kollman, "Die Grippe in Java in Jahre 1831," *Hecker's Wissenschaftl. Annalen der Geschichte Heilkunde* 26 (1833): 389.

20. Ibid., 389–90; and T. M. Ward, "An Account of the Epidemic of Catarrh, Which Prevailed at Penang in July and August 1831," *Transactions of the Medical and Physical Society of Calcutta* 6 (1833), 131–33. Ward cites an article in a Dutch colonial newspaper.

21. Ward, "Catarrh Which Prevailed at Penang," 124–35.

22. Ann Jannetta, personal communication, 26 June 1985.

23. Unless otherwise noted, European data are from Gluge, *Die Influ-*

enza, 136–37; Schweich, Die Influenza, 22–23; Hirsch, Handbook, vol. 1, 13; and Ripperger, Die Influenza, 81–84.

24. Von Stosch, "Die Influenza-Epidemieen in Berlin in den Jahren 1831 und 1833," Wochenschrift für die gesammte Heilkunde (Berlin) 1 (1833): 449.

25. Axel Petersen, "Feberaaret 1831," Ugeskrift fur Laeger 94 (14 January 1932): 54; A. F. Bremer and E. Fenger, "Om Influenza-Epidemierne i Danmark i Aarene 1825 till 1844," Kongelige Medicinske Selskabs Skrifter (Copenhagen) (1848): 213.

26. John Burne, "The Present Influenza," London Medical Gazette 8 (1831): 430.

27. J. Anderson, "Some Account of an Epidemic Influenza Which Prevailed in Glasgow May Last," Glasgow Medical Examiner 1 (1831–32): 89.

28. Guerin, "L'épidémie de Paris," 217.

29. Lombard, "Grippe qui a régné à Genève," 729.

30. Giacomo Folchi, "Relazione della malattia reumatico catarrh distinta dai Francesi col nome Grippe, che ha dominato in Roma sul finir dell'anno 1831," Bolletino delle scienze mediche (Bologna): 5 (1832): 115.

31. Porter, An Account of the Origin, 31.

32. Daniel Drake, "Notices of the Influenza and Measles as They Appeared at Cincinnati, in 1831–2," Western Journal of Medicine and Physical Science 6 (Cincinnati, 1833): 45–46.

33. Porter, An Account of the Origin, 13.

34. A. C. Baldwin, "Influenza of 1831–32 as it appeared in Burke County," 30. Burke County is south of Augusta on the South Carolina border.

35. Porter, An Account of the Origin, 9.

36. S. Ludlow, "Brief Notice of a Mild Epidemic Fever Which Prevailed at Indore and Other Parts of India, in April, 1832," Transactions of the Medical and Physical Society of Calcutta 6 (1833): 473–74.

37. George Playfair, "On the Epidemic Fever Which Prevailed in the Merut Division," Transactions of the Medical and Physical Society of Calcutta 6 (1833): 474.

38. Hirsch, Handbook, vol. 1, 14.

39. Bennett, "Influenza . . . at Manila," 524; Ward, "Catarrh Which Prevailed at Penang," 132.

40. Kollman, "Die Grippe in Java," 396–97.

41. Joseph J.-N. Fuster, Monographie clinique de l'affection catarrhale (Montpellier, France, 1861), 434.

42. Lombard, "Grippe qui a régné à Genève," 729–30.

43. Chevally, "Note sur l'épidémie qui a régné à Naples en 1833," Gazette médicale de Paris, 2d sér., vol. 2 (1833): 252.

44. Charles Creighton, A History of Epidemics in Britain, 2d ed., vol. 2 (New York, 1965), 379–80.

45. Anderson, "Influenza Which Prevailed at Glasgow," 91.

46. Lemuel Shattuck, "On the Vital Statistics of Boston," American Journal of the Medical Sciences," n.s., vol. 1 (1841): 377, 397. Cholera was also responsible for many "excess" deaths.

47. Burne, "The Present Influenza," 430; Lombard, "Grippe qui a régné à Genève," 730.

48. D. Finkler, "Influenza," in *Twentieth Century Practice: An International Encyclopedia of Modern Medical Science*, vol. 15 (New York, 1898), 38, suggests that the pandemic reached French Guiana in early 1834, but his source is cryptic and the idea seems extremely doubtful. See Segond, "Compte-rendu de la clinique médico-chirurgicale de Cayenne," *Journal Hebdomadaire des progrès des sciences et institutions médicales* 1 (1835): 354.

49. A. C. Kusnezow and F. L. Herrmann, *Influenza: Eine geschichtliche und klinesche Studie* (Vienna, 1890; trans. from Russian by J. V. Drozda), 31; M. Webster Brown, "Early Epidemics of Influenza in America," *Medical Journal and Record* 135 (4 May 1932): 449; Beveridge, *Influenza*, 29.

50. Unless otherwise cited, data are derived from Schweich, *Die Influenza*. 24; Gluge, *Die Influenza oder Grippe*, 144–146; Hirsch, *Handbook*, vol. 1, 14; Ripperger, *Die Influenza*, 91–92.

51. C. W. H. Ronander, "Något om den nu gångbara Influenza," *Tidskrift för Läkare och pharmaceuter* 2 (1833): 201.

52. C. W. Hufeland, "Die diesjährige Influenza," *Journal der practischen Heilkunde* 3 (1833): 119–20.

53. Bremer and Fenger, "Om Influenza-Epidemierne i Danmark," 214.

54. Hingeston, "On the Late Influenza," 199.

55. F. A. B. Puchelt, "Die Influenza, Grippe, im Jahre 1833," *Medizinische Annalen Heidelberg* 1 (1835): 549; C. Trafvenfeldt, "Influenza år 1833," *Tidskrift för Läkare och Pharmaceuter* 3 (1834): 275.

56. Giovanni Cavina, *L'influenza epidemica attraverso i secoli* (Rome, 1959), 169.

57. Blosch, "Einege Bemerkungen über Katarralfieberepidemien im bernischen Seelande," *Schweitzerische Zeitschrift für Medizin, Chirurgie und Geburtschirugie* 4 (1848): 324.

58. Domenico Sorrettone, "Storia della febbere catarrale epidemica regnata in Pozzuoli nel mese di novembre dell' anno 1833," *Esculapio Napolitano* 85 (1834): 5.

59. Hufeland, *Die diesjährige Influenza*, 119.

60. Ronander, "Gångbara Influenza," 203.

61. Brown, "Influenza in Edinburgh," 27.

62. Fuster, *Monographie clinique*, 440.

63. Creighton, *Epidemics in Britain*, vol. 2, 381.

64. Ripperger, *Die Influenza*, 88.

65. A. Brierre de Boismont, *Considérations pratiques sur la grippe, son histoire, sa nature, et son traitement* (Paris, 1833), 14.

66. Ronander, "Gångbara Influenza," 203; R. Venables, "Remarks on the Influenza or Catarrhal Epidemic of 1833," *Lancet* 2 (1833): 201.

67. Gluge, *Die Influenza oder Grippe*, 142–43.

68. Ripperger, *Die Influenza*, 88.

69. Brown, "Influenza in Edinburgh," 30.

70. Creighton, *Epidemics in Britain*, vol. 2, 383.

71. E. A. Wrigley and R. S. Schofield, *The Population History of England, 1541–1871* (Cambridge, Mass., 1981), 337–38.

72. Fyfe, *Observations on Influenza*, 3.

73. Beveridge, *Influenza*, 65.

74. "The Influenza," *London Medical Gazette* 20 (1837): 129.

75. E. Brande, "Breaking Out of the Influenza at Cape Town," *London Medical Gazette* 20 (1837): 115.

76. Hirsch, *Handbook*, vol. 1, 14.

77. Henry Holland, *Medical Notes and Reflections*, 3d ed. (London, 1855), 328.

78. Unless otherwise noted, data are from Gluge, *Die Influenza oder Grippe*, 164–65; Hirsch, *Handbook*, vol. 1, 14–15; and Ripperger, *Die Influenza*, 98–99.

79. Bremer and Fenger, "Om Influenza-Epidemierne i Danmark," 215.

80. M. Pétrequin, "Recherches pour servir à l'histoire générale de la grippe de 1837 en France et en Italie," *Gazette médicale de Paris*, 2d sér., 5 (1837): 803. See also F.-J. Malcorps, *La grippe et ses épidémies; ou recherches historiques, théoretiques et pratiques sur cette maladie* (Brussels, 1874), 19.

81. Klas Linroth, C. Wallis, and F. W. Warfvinge, *Influenza in Svedig* (Stockholm, 1890), vi–vii.

82. Marc D'Espine, "De la grippe à Genève en 1848," *Gazette médicale de Paris*, 3d sér., 3 (1848): 372; Lombard, "Note sur l'épidémie de grippe qui a régné à Genève en février 1837," *Gazette médicale de Paris*, 2d sér., 5 (1837): 214.

83. Lima Leitão, "Noticia acerca da grippe qui tem grassado em Lisboa desde o meio de fevereiro de corrente anno," *Jornal da Sociedade de ciencias medicas de Lisboa* 5 (1837): 20, 37.

84. Cavina, *L'influenza epidemica*, 175.

85. Holland, *Medical Notes*, 328.

86. John Hjaltelin, "On the Epidemic Influenzas of Iceland, Especially the Last One of 1862," *Edinburgh Medical Journal* 8 (1863): 698.

87. Pétrequin, "Recherches," 802–3; Lombard, "Note sur l'épidémie," 216.

88. Henry Bullock, "Influenza: Nature and Treatment of the Present Epidemic," *London Medical Gazette* 19 (1837): 700.

89. D'Espine, "De la grippe à Genève," 373.

90. Gluge, *Die Influenza oder Grippe*, 170.

91. Lombard, "Note sur l'épidémie," 214.

92. Pétrequin, "Recherches," 805.

93. Robert Streeten, "Report on the Influenza or Epidemic Catarrh of the Winter of 1836–37," (1838), in Thompson, *Annals*, 310.

94. R. J. Graves, "On the Influenza," *London Medical Gazette* 20 (1837): 787–88.

95. Legrande, "Note pour servir à l'histoire de la grippe en Paris," *Gazette médicale de Paris*, 2d sér., 5 (1837): 137.

96. L. Landau. "Mémoire sur la grippe de 1837, et sur la pneumonie considerée comme symptôme essentiel de cette épidémie," *Archives générales de médecine* (Paris), 2d sér., 13 (1837): 433–34.

97. John Clendinning, "Notice of the Influenza of January and February, 1837," *London Medical Gazette* 19 (1837): 781–82.

98. Gluge, *Die Influenza*, 160.

99. Linroth, *Influenza in Svedig*, vii.

100. D'Espine, "De la grippe à Genève," 387.

101. Creighton, *Epidemics in Britain*, vol. 2, 386.

102. Streeten, "Report on the Influenza," 303.

103. Graves, "On the Influenza," 787–88; D'Espine, "De la grippe à Genève," 387; Landau, "Mémoire sur la grippe de 1837," 444–45.

104. H. Wakefield, "Influenza as It Prevailed in the House of Correction," *London Medical Gazette* 19 (1837): 705.

105. Hirsch, *Handbook*, vol. 1, 16.

106. Ibid.

107. Luther H. Gulick, "On the Climate, Diseases, and Materia Medica of the Sandwich (Hawaiian) Islands," *New York Journal of Medicine* 14 (1855): 14.

108. Unless otherwise noted, data from Hirsch, *Handbook*, vol. 1, 16; Ripperger, *Die Influenza*, 100–104; and Finkler, "Influenza," 41.

109. H. Theilmann, "Die Influenza in St. Petersburg im Marz und April 1847," *Medizinische Zeiting Russlands* 4 (1847): 147.

110. André Leval, "Lettre sur le Cholera qui règne actuellement à Constantinople," *Gazette médicale de Paris*, 3d sér., 2 (1847): 1009; Thomas B. Peacock, *On the Influenza or Epidemic Catarrhal Fever of 1847–8* (London, 1848), 12.

111. Cavina, *L'influenza epidemica*, 189; *Annual Report of the Registrar General of Births, Deaths, and Marriages in England* 10 (1847), xxxi.

112. *Det Kongelige Sundhedskollegiums Forhandlinger*, 1847, 10.

113. *Gazzetta Medica Lombarda*, 7 Feb. 1848, 68.

114. D'Espine, "De la grippe à Genève," 373.

115. "Noticia sobre la grippe en Madrid," *Boletin de Medicina, Cirugia y Farmacia* (Madrid), 3 (1848): 19.

116. *Gazzetta Medica Lombarda*, 10 Jan. 1848, 24.

117. Ibid., 31 Jan. 1848, 58.

118. Blösch, "Einige Bemerkungen," 327.

119. *Det Kongelige Sundhedskollegiums Forhandlinger*, 1848, 11; Hjaltelin, "Epidemic Influenzas of Iceland," 698.

120. Linroth, *Influenza in Svedig*, vii.

121. Fuster, *Monographie clinique*, 473.

122. See also Pyle and Patterson, "Influenza Diffusion in European History," 176–77.

123. Peacock, *On the Influenza . . . of 1847–48*, 13.

124. D'Espine, "De la grippe à Genève," 373.

125. Ripperger, *Die Influenza*, 101.

126. Fuster, *Monographie clinique*, 473, 477.

127. D'Espine, "De la grippe à Genève," 386–88.

128. Malcorps, *La grippe et ses épidémies*, 21.

129. *Registrar General's Report* (Great Britain) 10 (1847): xxviii–xxx.

130. H. Franklin Parsons, "The Influenza Epidemics of 1889–90 and 1891, and Their Distribution in England and Wales," *British Medical Journal*, 8 August 1891, 303.

131. Among those who have described 1847–48 as a true pandemic are

Warren T. Vaughan, *Influenza: An Epidemiologic Survey* (Baltimore, 1921),
12; G. C. Schild, "Influenza," in *A World Geography of Human Diseases*, ed.
G. Melvyn Howe (London and New York, 1977), 365; Brown, "Early Epi-
demics of Influenza in America," 449; Hirsch, *Handbook*, vol. 1, 18; and
Pyle and Patterson, "Influenza Diffusion in European History," 180. Edwin
D. Kilbourne, "Epidemiology of Influenza," in *The Influenza Viruses and
Influenza*, ed. Kilbourne (New York, 1975), 494, is more cautious.
    132. Hirsch, *Handbook*, vol. 1, 17; Ripperger, *Die Influenza*, 105–6.
    133. Beveridge, *Influenza*, 30.
    134. Pyle and Patterson, "Influenza in European History," 182–83.

Chapter 4

    1. Partial exceptions include Bremer and Fenger on Denmark and the
Registrar-General's Report of 1847 for England and Wales, both cited in
chapter 3.
    2. Questionnaire responses were used in official reports by H. F. Par-
sons in *Report on the Influenza Epidemic of 1889–90*. Local Government
Board (London, 1891), published in *Parliamentary Papers*, Cmd. 6387
(1891); and J. K. A. Wertheim Salomonson and C. de Rooij, "Rapport over de
Influenza-epidemic in Nederland van 1889–90," *Nederlandsch Tijdschrift
voor Geneeskunde*, 2R, 29, pt. 2 (1893), 688–778. An example of such a
report sponsored by a medical society is Raoul Brunon, *Rapport sur la
marche de l'épidémie de grippe dans la Seine-Inférieure pendant les mois
de novembre-decembre 1889 et janvier-février 1890* (Rouen, 1890).
    3. Charles Creighton, the English epidemiologist, remained a staunch
miasmatist even after the pandemic. J. Tessier, *L'influenza de 1889–1890 en
Russie* (Paris, 1891), explained the origins of the pandemic in terms reminiscent of Max von Pettenkofer's groundwater theories. Miasmatic views were
still common in Britain, as seen in a survey by Parsons, *Report*, 121–51; and
in France, Vergely, *Rapport sur l'épidémie de grippe ou influenza qui a sévi
en 1889–90 dans le département de la Gironde* (Bordeaux, 1891), 8.
    4. See, for example, O. Leichtenstern, "Influenza," in *Malaria, Influ-
enza, and Dengue*, ed. Julius Mannaberg and O. Leichtenstern (Philadelphia, 1905), 538–40; and Richard Sisley, *Epidemic Influenza: Notes on Its
Origin and Method of Spread* (London, 1891), 33–36.
    5. I am grateful to Dr. Frank Barrett of York University, Ontario, for
confirming this in a personal communication of 22 August 1985. Dr. Barrett
is working on a history of medical geography.
    6. A. Ripperger, *Die Influenza: Ihre Geschichte, Epidemiologie,
Aetiologie, Symptomatologie and Therapie* (Munich, 1892), 106–7; August
Hirsch, *Handbook of Geographical and Historical Pathology*, vol. 1 (Lon-
don, 1883), 17–18.
    7. Ripperger, *Die Influenza*, 107.
    8. Frank Clemow, "The Recent Pandemic of Influenza: Its Place of
Origin and Mode of Spread," pt. 1, *Lancet* (20 Jan. 1894): 140.
    9. Parsons, *Report*, 9.
    10. Ibid., 14; Leichtenstern, "Influenza," 534; F. M. Burnet and E. Clarke,

Influenza: A Survey of the Last Fifty Years in the Light of Modern Work on the Virus of Epidemic Influenza (Melbourne, 1942), 61; C. Stuart-Harries, "Pandemic Influenza: An Unresolved Problem in Prevention," *Journal of Infectious Diseases* 122 (1970): 110; W. I. B. Beveridge, *Influenza: The Last Great Plague: An Unfinished Story of Discovery* (New York, 1977), 30.

11. I have not been able to consult Heyfelder's original clinical description, but extensive excerpts and discussion are given in Sisley, *Epidemic Influenza*, 48–50; Tessier, *L'influenza en Russie*, 48–49; and in Warren T. Vaughan, *Influenza: An Epidemiologic Study* (Baltimore, 1921), 15. Heyfelder published his later views in "Zu den Epidemien von 1889," *St. Petersburger Medicinische Wochenschrift* 15 (1890): 87–88.

12. Parsons, *Report*, 9.

13. Julius Althaus, *Influenza; Its Pathology, Symptoms, Complications, and Sequels; Its Origin and Mode of Spreading: and Its Diagnosis, Prognosis, and Treatment*, 2d ed. (London, 1892), 315–20.

14. Clemow, "The Recent Pandemic," 140, n. 10.

15. Tessier, *L'influenza en Russie*, 49.

16. Ripperger, *Die Influenza*, 109–10.

17. James Cantlie, "The First Recorded Appearance of the Modern Influenza Epidemic," *British Medical Journal* 2 (29 August 1891): 491.

18. Clemow, "The Recent Pandemic," 143.

19. Clemow, "Epidemic Influenza," *Public Health* (U.K.) 2 (April 1890): 361–65.

20. Clemow, "The Recent Pandemic," pt. 1, 139–43; and pt. 2, *Lancet* (10 February 1894): 329–31. His views are restated in the chapter on influenza in *The Geography of Disease* (Cambridge, 1903), 187–203. Clemow's use of the Old Style (Julian) dates then employed in Russia has caused some confusion in the secondary literature.

21. Tessier, *L'influenza en Russie*, 2–4, 10–14.

22. Losch, "Notice sur l'épidémie d'influenza à Kief, en 1889," *Province médicale* (Lyon) 5 (1891): 157–60.

23. Klas Linroth, C. Wallis, and F. W. Warfvinge, *Influenza in Svedig* (Stockholm, 1890), 3–17 and map.

24. Jacques Bertillon, *La grippe à Paris et dans quelques autres villes de France et de l'étranger en 1889–90* (Paris, 1892), 102.

25. See, for example, Tessier, *L'influenza en Russie*, map opp. p. 38; Althaus, *Influenza*, 290–92; A. Proust, "Sur l'enquête concernant l'épidémie de grippe de 1889–90 en France," *Bulletin de l'académie de médecine de Paris*, 3d sér., 27 (1892), 523–25; and A. Villard, *Leçons cliniques à propos de l'épidémie de 1889 et 1890* (Paris, 1890), 109–11. Unless otherwise noted, data are from Ripperger, *Die Influenza*; Parsons, *Report*; and Lechtenstern, "Influenza."

26. A. Ulrick, "Den Danske Faellesforskning angaaende Influenza-Epidemien," *Bibliot. f. Laeger* 1 (1890): 474–75.

27. Linroth, *Influenza in Svedig*, map and 4–5.

28. F. Schmid, *Die Influenza in der Schweitz 1889–1894* (Berne, 1895), map 1.

29. Wertheim Salmonson and de Rooij, "Influenza-epidemie in Nederland," 690–97.

30. Overviews of the situation in France are given in Proust, "Sur l'enquête," 510–31, 552–96; and Victor Turquan, "Statistiques des épidémies de grippe de 1890 et 1892 en France," *Journal de la société de statistique de Paris* 34 (1893): 60–66, 80–98.

31. Brunon, *Grippe dans la Seine-Inférieure*, 7–8.

32. J. M. Durand, "Histoire de l'épidémie de grippe à Bordeaux," *Mémoires and Bulletin de la société de médecine et chirurgie de Bordeaux* (1891), 71–72.

33. H. Alezias, "Rapport sur l'épidémie de grippe à Marseille, pendant l'hiver 1889–90," *Marseille médicale* 27 (1890): 622.

34. This lag is evident in the mortality data presented in Turquan, "Statistiques," 90–93.

35. Alfonso Corradi, "L'influenza in Italia nel 1890," *Gazzeta medica Lombarda* 50 (1890): 391.

36. Silva Carvalho, "Estudos portuguêzes acerca da grippe: A pandemia de influenza em Lisboa," *A Medicina Contemporanea* 8 (1890): 105; Alberto Antonio de Moraes Carvalho Sabrinho, Virgilio Machado, Alfredo Luiz Lopes, and Gregorio Rodrigues Fernandes, "Relatorio sobre a epidemia qui em Lisboa grassou desde dezembro de 1889 até fevereiro de 1890," *A Medicina Contemporânea* 8 (1890): 132.

37. L. G. Limarakis, "L'épidémie de grippe influenza à Constantinople," *Revue médico-pharmaceutique de Constantinople* 3 (1890): 9, 74–76; Althaus, *Influenza*, 291–92.

38. Parsons, "The Influenza Epidemics of 1889–90 and 1891, and Their Distribution in England and Wales," *British Medical Journal* (8 Aug. 1891): 305.

39. John W. Moore, "The Influenza Epidemic of 1889–90 as Observed in Dublin," *Dublin Journal of Medical Sciences* 89 (1890): 301.

40. Parsons, "The Influenza Epidemics," 305.

41. Andrew Dunlop, "On Influenza in Jersey," *Glasgow Medical Journal* 33 (1890): 416–19; John Aikman, "Influenza in Guernsey, 1890," *Glasgow Medical Journal* 33 (1890): 411–12.

42. For example, Parsons, "The Influenza Epidemics," 305; Althaus, *Influenza*, 295; Proust, "Sur l'enquête," 528; Turquan, "Statistiques," 773; Brunon, "Grippe dans la Seine-Inférieure," 7–8.

43. Linroth, *Influenza in Svedig*; Wertheim Salmonson and de Rooij, "Influenza-epidemie in Nederland"; Schmid, *Influenza in der Schweitz*.

44. Paul L. Friedrich, *Die Influenza-Epidemie 1889–1890 im Deutschen Reiche*, in *Arbeiten aus dem Kaiserlichen Gesundheitamte*, vol. 9 (1894), table 10, map.

45. Schmid, *Influenza in der Schweitz*, map 1.

46. Althaus, *Influenza*, 303–6.

47. Antonio Mora, *La epidemia d'influenza nella provincia di Bergamo nell'anno 1890* (Bergamo, Italy, 1890), 7–12 and map.

48. Unless otherwise cited, data are from Parsons, *Report*; Ripperger, *Die Influenza*; and Leichtenstern, "Influenza."

49. *Virginia Medical Monthly*, "Influenza Epidemic of 1890 as it Occurred in Richmond" 16 (1889–90): 978.

50. Yates Trotter, Jr., "The Influenza Epidemic of 1889–90," U.S. Com-

municable Disease Center, Influenza Surveillance Report no. 21, appendix B, 15 October 1957 (Atlanta), 2.

51. Trotter, "Epidemic of 1889–90," 2.

52. Unless otherwise cited, data are from Parsons, *Report;* Ripperger, *Die Influenza;* and Leichtenstern, "Influenza."

53. G. Mendizabal, "Contribución al estudio de la gripa en Mexico," *Gaceta médica de Mexico* 36 (1899): 349–50.

54. M. Amaral, "La influenza en Santiago," *Revista médica de Chile* 19 (1890–91): 92.

55. Amaral, "La influenza," 92.

56. Jose C. Ulloa, "La grippe del Peru," *El Monitor Médico* (Lima) 5 (15 April 1890): 337.

57. Ulrick, "Den Danske," 472.

58. Unless otherwise cited, data are from Parsons, *Report;* Ripperger, *Die Influenza;* and Leichtenstern, "Influenza."

59. Franz Engel Bey, *L'épidémie d'influenza en Egypte pendant l'hiver 1889–1890,* Egypt, Administration des Services sanitaires et d'hygiène publique (Cairo, 1894), 5–12 and map.

60. William C. Scholtz, "The Influenza Epidemic at the Cape," *British Medical Journal* 1 (1890): 600.

61. B. W. Quartey-Papafio, "The Epidemic of Influenza," *Lancet* (13 December 1890): 1302. Elmina was also attacked in April.

62. W. T. Prout, "The Epidemic of Influenza," *Lancet* (16 August 1890): 370–71. Cape Coast and Axim were also attacked in May.

63. John Bowie, "Influenza and Ear Disease in Central Africa," *Lancet* (11 July 1891): 66–68.

64. J.-D. Tholozan, "La grippe en Perse en 1889–90," *Bulletin de l'Académie de Médecine de Paris,* 3d sér., 26 (1891), 256–58. Unless otherwise cited, data are from Parsons, *Report;* Ripperger, *Die Influenza;* and Leichtenstern, "Influenza."

65. Engel Bey, *Influenza en Egypt,* 5.

66. Kailas C. Bose, "Influenza as Seen in Calcutta, and Its Treatment," *Indian Medical Gazette* 25 (1890): 181.

67. James M. MacPhail, "The Influenza Epidemic in Rural Bengal," *Glasgow Medical Journal* 34 (1890): 187.

68. Cantlie, "The First Recorded Appearance," 491.

69. K. Ci-Min Wong and Wu Lien-teh, *History of Chinese Medicine,* 2d ed. (Shanghai, 1936), 837. The table of epidemics cited has no influenza entry for 1888–1889, but does have entries for 1890 and 1891.

70. Cantlie, "The First Recorded Appearance," 491.

71. Parsons, *Report,* 41.

72. Leichtenstern, "Influenza," 594.

73. J. C. Verco, "The Epidemic of Influenza in Adelaide in 1890," *Australian Medical Gazette* 9 (1889–90): 221.

74. Clemow, "The Recent Pandemic," 329 and map, 140.

75. Proust, "Sur l'enquête," 523–25; Tessier, *L'influenza en Russie,* map opp. p. 38; and Bertillon, *La grippe à Paris,* map.

76. Turquan, "Statistiques," 83–96.

77. Leichtenstern, "Influenza," 545.

78. Ibid., 545–48.

79. H. Franklin Parsons, *Further Reports and Papers on Epidemic Influenza, 1889–1892*, Local Government Board (London, 1893), published in Parliamentary Papers, Cmd. 7051, 1893.

80. Leichtenstern, "Influenza," 551–53.

81. Parsons, *Further Reports*, 50–53.

82. Vaughan, *Influenza*, 44–45.

83. Mora, *Influenza nella provincia di Bergamo*, 14–17.

84. Leichtenstern, "Influenza," 570–72; Vaughan, *Influenza*, 148–50.

85. Leichtenstern, "Influenza," 570–71.

86. Schmid, *Influenza in der Schweitz*, presents graphs for nine cantons in table 3.

87. Turquan, "Statistiques," 64–65.

88. Leichtenstern, "Influenza," 568.

89. Wertheim Salmonson and de Rooij, "Influenza-epidemie in Nederland," 753–55.

90. F. A. Dixey, *Epidemic Influenza: A Study in Comparative Statistics* (London, 1892), 23.

91. Bertillon, *La grippe à Paris*, 102.

92. Silva Carvalho, "Estudos portuguêzes acerca da grippe," 173.

93. Bertillon, *La grippe à Paris*, 125 and map.

94. Turquan, "Statistiques," 95–96.

95. Parsons, *Further Reports*," 3–5.

96. Bertillon, *La grippe à Paris*, map.

97. Great Britain, Ministry of Health, *Report on the Pandemic of Influenza, 1918–1919* (London, 1920), 21–27.

98. Dixey, *Epidemic Influenza*, 23.

99. Great Britain, *Report on the Pandemic*, 52.

100. Losch, "Influenza à Kief," 157–59.

101. Bowie, "Influenza in Central Africa," 68.

102. Oluf Thomsen, M. Kristensen, and F. Thorborg, *Undersgelser over Influenza ens (den "spanske sypes") aarsagsforhold* (Copenhagen, 1918), 9.

103. Engel Bey, *Influenza en Egypte*, tables, 37.

104. Great Britain, *Report on the Pandemic*, 31–34.

105. It is, for example, not listed by Beveridge, *Influenza*; or G. C. Schild, "Influenza," in *A World Geography of Human Disease* ed. G. Melvyn Howe (London and New York, 1977), 365; or Vaughan, *Influenza*, 12. Edwin D. Kilbourne did include 1900 in his list of pandemics in "Influenza Pandemics in Perspective," *Journal of the American Medical Association* 237 (21 March 1977): 1225. There is, however, general recognition that there was a fair amount of influenza around this time.

106. Robert J. Wolfe, "Alaska's Great Sickness, 1900: An Epidemic of Measles and Influenza in a Virgin Soil Population," *Proceedings of the American Philosophical Society* 126, no. 2 (1982): 91–121.

107. *Public Health Reports* 16 (1901): 874.

108. Announcements in *Lancet* 2 (1899): 1753; *Lancet* 1 (1900): 67, 107, 135, 181, 201; and in *British Medical Journal* 1 (1900): 36, 97, 150, 238, 362.

109. A. Giltray, "De Influenza-Epidemie te Amsterdam, Vergeleken met die van 1890 en 1900," *Nederlansch Tijdschrift voor Geneeskunde* 61 (23 November 1918): 1678; Thomsen et al., *Undersgelser over Influenza*, 6.

110. *Lancet* 1 (1900): 274–75, 349–50.

111. *Bulletin de l'Académie de Médecine* 43 (1900): 301; Condamy, "Notes sur l'épidémie de grippe de 1899–1900," *Bulletin de la Société de médecine et chirurgie de La Rochelle* 32 (1900): 127–30.

112. J. B. Busdraghi, "La influenza en Madrid: profilaxis y traitamiento," *La Correspondencia médica* 36 (1901): 184.

113. R. R. Stawell, "A Note on Influenza in Children, With Special Reference to Unusual Cases," *International Medical Journal of Australasia* (20 Nov. 1901): 525.

114. See further discussion in chapter 5.

Chapter 5

1. Gerald F. Pyle and K. David Patterson, "Influenza Diffusion in European History: Patterns and Paradigms," *Ecology of Disease* 2 (1984): 173–84.

2. See, for example, A. Villard, *Leçons cliniques à propos de l'épidémie de 1889 et 1890* (Paris, 1890), 106–8.

3. John Norris, "East or West? The Geographic Origin of the Black Death," *Bulletin of the History of Medicine* 51 (1977): 8.

4. C. A. Gill, *The Genesis and Natural History of Disease* (New York, 1928), 223.

5. C. H. Andrewes, "Asiatic Influenza: A Challenge to Epidemiology," in *Perspectives in Virology*, ed. M. Pollard (1959): 185–86.

6. W. I. B. Beveridge, *Influenza: The Last Great Plague: An Unfinished Story of Discovery* (New York, 1978), 40, 42.

7. W. G. Laver and R. G. Webster, "Ecology of Influenza Viruses in Lower Animals and Birds," *British Medical Bulletin* 35 (1979): 32; R. G. Webster, W. G. Laver, G. M. Air, and G. C. Schild, "Molecular Mechanisms of Variation in Influenza Viruses," *Nature* 296 (11 Mar. 1982): 117; Guo Yuanji, Wang Min, Jin Fengen, Wing Ping and Zhu Jiming, "Influenza Ecology in China," in *The Origin of Pandemic Influenza Viruses*, ed. W. G. Laver (New York, 1983), 211.

8. R. G. Webster, W. G. Laver, and C. M. Chu, "Summary of a Meeting on the Origin of Pandemic Influenza Viruses," *Journal of Infectious Diseases* 149 (Jan. 1984): 108–15; K. F. Shortridge, "Pandemic Influenza: Application of Epidemiology and Ecology in the Region of Southern China to Prospective Studies," in *Origin of Pandemic Influenza Viruses*, ed. Laver, 191–200; Shortridge and C. H. Stuart-Harries, "An Influenza Epicentre?" *Lancet* 2 (9 Oct. 1982): 812–13.

9. Laver and Webster, "Ecology of Influenza Viruses," 32.

10. A. P. Kendal, G. R. Noble, J. J. Skehel, and W. R. Dowdle, "Antigenic Similarity of Influenza A (H1N1) Viruses from Epidemic of 1977–1978 to 'Scandinavian' Strains Isolated in Epidemics of 1950–51," *Virology* 274 (1978): 633; R. Palese and C. Brand, "Molecular Epidemiology of Influenza

Viruses," in *Perspectives in Virology*, vol. 11, ed. M. Pollard (1981), 115–27, including discussion.

11. Norris, "East or West?" 1–2. His views on plague are still being debated.

12. Beveridge, *Influenza*, 91–92.

13. Pyle and Patterson, "Influenza Diffusion in European History," 182–83.

14. Beveridge, *Influenza*, 49–51.

15. W. P. Glezen, R. B. Couch, and H. R. Six, "The Influenza Herald Wave," *American Journal of Epidemiology* 116 (Oct. 1982): 589–98.

16. F. L. Dunn, "Pandemic Influenza in 1957: Review of International Spread of New Asian Strain," *Journal of the American Medical Association (JAMA)* 166 (8 Mar. 1958): 1140–48; A. D. Langmuir, "Epidemiology of Asian Influenza, With Special Emphasis on the United States," *American Review of Respiratory Diseases* 83 (1961): 2–14; E. D. Kilbourne, "Epidemiology of Influenza," in *The Influenza Viruses and Influenza*, ed. Kilbourne (New York, 1975), 498–502.

17. V. S. Hinshaw and R. G. Webster, "The Natural History of Influenza A Viruses," in *Basic and Applied Influenza Research*, ed. A. S. Beare (Boca Raton, Fla., 1982), 79–104; D. J. Alexander, "Ecological Aspects of Influenza A Viruses in Animals and Their Relationship to Human Influenza: A Review," *Journal of the Royal Society of Medicine* 75 (Oct. 1982): 799–811.

18. A. Hirsch, *Handbook of Geographical and Historical Pathology*, vol. 1 (London, 1883), 38–39.

19. J. Arbuthnot, "An Essay Concerning the Effects of Air on the Human Body" (London, 1751), in *Annals of Influenza or Epidemic Catarrhal Fever in Great Britain from 1510 to 1837*, ed. T. Thompson (London, 1852), 38.

20. A. Fothergill, "An Account of Epidemic Catarrh (Termed Influenza) as It Appeared at Northampton . . . ," *Memoirs of the Medical Society of London* 3 (1792): 34–35.

21. T. Glass, in Thompson, *Annals of Influenza*, 102; R. Pultney, in ibid., 112.

22. B. Parr, "An Account of the Influenza, as it Appeared in Devonshire in May 1782," *Medical Commentaries* 5 (1783–85): 257.

23. B. Rush, "An Account of the Influenza as It Appeared in Philadelphia in the Autumn of 1789, in the Spring of 1790, and in the Winter of 1791," in his *Medical Inquiries and Observations*, 3d ed., vol. 2 (Philadelphia, 1809), 446.

24. Thompson, *Annals of Influenza*, 213–14.

25. T. M. Ward, "An Account of the Epidemic of Catarrh, Which Prevailed at Penang, in July and August 1831," *Transactions of the Medical and Physical Society of Calcutta* 6 (1833), 126.

26. Youatt, in Thompson, *Annals of Influenza*, 291.

27. Thompson, *Annals of Influenza*, 361.

28. M. Pétrequin, "Recherches pour servir à l'histoire générale de la grippe de 1837 en France et in Italie," *Gazette médicale de Paris*, 2d sér., 5 (1837): 805.

29. R. Sisley, *Epidemic Influenza: Notes on its Origin and Method of Spread* (London, 1891), 117–30; E. Symes-Thompson, *Influenza or Epi-*

demic Catarrhal Fever: An Historical Survey of Past Epidemics in Great Britain From 1510 to 1890 (London, 1890), 419–21; O. Leichtenstern, "Influenza," in Malaria, Influenza, and Dengue, eds. J. Mannaberg and O. Leichtenstern (Philadelphia, 1905), 587. For a recent discussion, see B. C. Easterday, "Animal Influenza," in Kilbourne, Influenza, 449–51.

30. Kilbourne, "Epidemiology of Influenza," 511.

31. R. E. Hope-Simpson, "Recognition of Historic Influenza Epidemics from Parish Burial Records: A Test of Prediction from a New Hypothesis of Influenzal Epidemiology," Journal of Hygiene 91 (Oct. 1983): 293–308.

32. E. A. Wrigley and R. S. Schofield, The Population History of England 1541–1871 (Cambridge, Mass., 1981), 332–33.

33. See, for example, Charles E. Rosenberg, The Cholera Years: The United States in 1832, 1849 and 1866 (Chicago, 1962); and Roderick E. McGrew, Russia and the Cholera 1823–1832 (Madison, Wis., 1965).

34. N. Masurel and R. A. Heijtink, "Recycling of H1N1 Influenza A Virus in Man—A Haemagglutinin Antibody Study," Journal of Hygiene 90 (1983): 397–402.

35. J. Mulder and N. Masurel, "Pre-Epidemic Antibody Against 1957 Strain of Asiatic Influenza in Serum of Older People Living in the Netherlands," Lancet (19 April 1958): 810–14; N. Masurel, "Serological Characteristics of a 'New' Serotype of Influenza A Virus: The Hong Kong Strain," Bulletin of the World Health Organization 41 (1969): 461–68; H. Fukumi, "Interpretation of Influenza Antibody Patterns in Man," Bulletin of the World Health Organization 41 (1969): 469–73; N. Masurel and W. M. Marine, "Recycling of Asian and Hong Kong Influenza A Virus Hemagglutinins in Man," American Journal of Epidemiology 97 (1973): 44–49; E. Kilbourne, "Influenza Pandemics in Perspective," JAMA 237 (21 Mar. 1977): 1226.

36. Gary R. Noble, "Epidemiological and Clinical Aspects of Influenza," in Basic and Applied Influenza Research, ed. Beare, 13.

37. Masurel and Heijtink, "Recycling of H1N1," 401; Masurel and Marine, "Recycling of Asian and Hong Kong Influenza A Viruses," 48; Masurel, "Swine Influenza Virus and the Recycling of Influenza-A Viruses in Man, Lancet (31 July 1976): 244.

38. Kilbourne, "Influenza Pandemics in Perspective," 1225 (11-year cycles); and Max Bader, "Influenza Cycles," JAMA 237 (17 June 1977): 2813 (68-year cycles).

39. Hope-Simpson, "Recognition of Historic Influenza Epidemics"; idem, "Epidemic Mechanisms of Type A Influenza," Journal of Hygiene 83 (1979): 11–26; idem, "The Role of Season in Epidemic Influenza," Journal of Hygiene 86 (1981): 35–47.

40. F. Hoyle and C. Wickramasinghe, "Does Epidemic Disease Come From Space?" New Scientist 76 (1977): 402–4.

Index